Advance P

"Highly recommended—practical guidance for everyday healthful living."
Joe Pizzorno, ND
Founding President, Bastyr University
Co-Author of *Encyclopedia of Natural Medicine*

"One of the most important steps you can take in the direction of abundant health is to carefully choose where you shop for food. It's a good idea, whenever possible, to shop at local farmer's markets, local natural food stores, or chains like Whole Foods and Wild Oats. And Larry Cook shows you how. As an introduction of many aspects of a natural lifestyle, his book makes it easy and fun to take care of yourself. Today's choices determine tomorrow's health."
–John Robbins, Author
Diet For A New America, The Food Revolution, Reclaiming Our Health

"*The Beginner's Guide to Natural Living* is the best first step anyone can take on the road to better living. Larry Cook has made simple the plan for changing the bad habits you didn't even realize you had. If you are interested in a long healthy life the best place to start is reading this book."
–Howard F. Lyman LL.D., Author
Mad Cowboy

"Where other health manuals fall short in over or underestimating their reader's knowledge of (and interest in) natural living, Larry offers readers a compelling introduction to the very idea of "natural living," avoiding common pitfalls like frightening statistics, unattainable goals or overly detailed descriptions of how to proceed.

Readers are introduced to adjunct ideas they may never have considered but which could play a role in either their illness or their recovery: holistic dentistry, internal acid-alkaline balance, genetically modified foods, even a short background on why natural therapies are effective and are therefore suppressed by the mainstream media and the conventional medical conglomerate.

I unreservedly recommend Larry Cook's guide to natural living as the perfect starting place for anyone seeking to improve their health and quality of life."
–Lori Lively, Director of Education
Marlene's Market & Deli; Tacoma, Washington

THE
Beginner's Guide to Natural Living

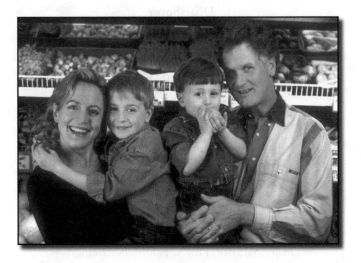

**How to cultivate a more natural lifestyle
to lose weight, prevent degenerative disease,
improve your energy and attain vibrant health.**

Larry Cook

EcoVision Communications

Los Angeles, CA

Publisher & Author's Web Site
www.TheNaturalGuide.com

Distributor
Book Publishing Company
PO Box 99
Summertown, TN 38483
888-260-8458

Writers
Larry Cook
Cynthia Logan

Editors
Kelley Guiney
Cynthia Logan

Foreword
Dr. John Taylor, Ph.D., Family Psychologist

Peer Reviews
Dr. Ron Hobbs, N.D., Bastyr University
Dr. John Taylor, Ph.D., Family Psychologist
Dr. Paul Rubin, DDS, Mercury Free Dentist

Photography & Cover Design
Larry Cook

Library of Congress Control Number
2005921811

ISBN 0-9755361-8-4 & 978-0-9755361-8-6

15 14 13 12 11 10   3 4 5 6 7 8 9 10

eBook Version

The *Beginner's Guide to Natural Living* is also available as a downloadable PDF file from the Internet. The eBook comes in two versions: "screen" and "print." The screen version is specifically formatted to be read on your computer screen, and throughout the eBook I include over 200 hyperlinks to a wide variety of Web sites for further study. The print version is specifically formatted to be printed, three hole punched and inserted into a binder. The pictures in the print version are in full color, and the pictures in the Appendix are twice the size as found in this softbound version. You may find the color pictures and larger format to be easier to use when shopping at the natural food store or preparing my meal suggestions. You can acquire the eBook by going to my Web site: **www.TheNaturalGuide.com**. Instructions for downloading and using the eBook are on the Web site.

Please Share With Me

Please let me know how *The Beginner's Guide to Natural Living* has helped you or changed your life; or let me know if you have any questions or feedback. My email is: **Larry@TheNaturalGuide.com**.

Disclaimer

The information presented in this book is not intended to diagnose, treat, cure or prevent any disease. The information contained herein is designed to educate the reader and is not intended to provide individual medical advice. If you have a medical condition, please consult a licensed health care practitioner.

Acknowledgments

The concept for this book—which has changed numerous times since I first conceived of it—may have been mine, but without the support and help of many people, this book would never have been created or be as accurate as possible. Therefore, a special thank you to the following people who have helped me make this book the best it could be:

Marilyn Frazier
Marilyn has been a steady support during the lows and highs of creating this book. Not only has she been emotionally supportive, but she invested her own money in its production because she believed in the project, and more importantly, she believed in me. Thank you, Marilyn.

Cynthia Logan
I met Cynthia in Bozeman, Montana shortly after I launched my first magazine devoted to natural living, and she worked for the magazine as a writer and editor. She rewrote several of my original pieces which I published as articles in my magazine, and which I collected and expanded in order to write this book. Cynthia edited and wrote several chapters of this book based on my input and research. There is simply no way I could have produced such excellent writing without Cynthia's intimate involvement with this project. Thank you, Cynthia.

Kelley Guiney
Kelley worked for me as a writer and editor when I launched my second magazine in Seattle. She has an amazing ability to really understand what I'm trying to say, and to help me say it clearly. She catches the smallest of details as well as the big ones, and her eagle eye helped make this book the best it could be. Thank you, Kelley.

Dr. Ron Hobbs, N.D.
Dr. Hobbs—a naturopathic physician and a faculty member at Bastyr University (Seattle, Washington)—reviewed the chapters that discuss detoxification, supplements and natural medicine. He gave invaluable

insight, clarified points and pointed out possible problem areas. His insights helped me to ensure that my information was as accurate as possible. Thank you, Dr. Hobbs.

Dr. John Taylor, Ph.D.
Dr. Taylor—a family psychologist and author of several books devoted to helping children with ADD/ADHD—not only reviewed my entire book and gave excellent feedback and editing, he wrote the Foreword as well! His feedback and editing suggestions were used throughout the book. Thank you, Dr. Taylor.

Dr. Paul Rubin, DDS
Dr. Rubin—a mercury free dentist in Seattle—helped me ensure that the dentistry chapter has the latest information. Thank you, Dr. Rubin.

Wild Oats Natural Food Store
Kristi Estes at the corporate Wild Oats ensured that I was able to shoot pictures at their Long Beach, California store. Employees and management at the store helped to ensure that I was able to shoot the best pictures possible. Not only did I wind up shooting great pictures for inside the book, but I shot an amazing photo to use on the front cover! Many thanks to Kristi Estes, staff at the Long Beach Wild Oats and corporate Wild Oats.

Special Thanks
Special thanks to Christine Forbing, Aileen Forbing, Patty Taulbee of PlantLife Natural Body Care, past advertisers and readers of my natural living magazines, Dan Poynter, author of *The Self-Publishing Manual*, Ganesh MacIsaac at Integral Yoga Distribution, Bob Holzapfel at the Book Publishing Company, Starr Bisonette of Nutri-Books, Lori Lively and Ashley Taulbee of Marlene's Market & Deli, Joe Delagarza, Lawrence Fried, my parents, my sister, and all who have supported me in writing, publishing and distributing my book.

Contents

Foreword
Dr. John Taylor, Ph.D.

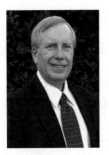

This book takes you on a journey to many unexpected places. It invites you to explore new ways of choosing what to eat and drink, where to shop for food, and even what to do for more meaningful and helpful recreation. Author Larry Cook is not intimidated by self-serving public relations blitzes from the food marketers, chemical companies, government bureaucracies, and agricultural industries that would mislead you about the food you're now eating and about its environmental impact. He tells you plainly and sincerely what works best for your total health—physically, mentally, and emotionally. This book is truly a guide to a new way of feeling better and living your life more productively.

He begins with water. You will learn how to obtain, purify, filter, restore, and conserve water for maximum benefit to your health and to Mother Earth. Next you'll learn about the more than 6000 "food cosmetic" chemicals that needlessly lace foods and beverages and how you can avoid their damaging effects. He shows you what to do about sugar and its substitutes and how to avoid unhealthy fats and oils.

Next, Larry takes you shopping, not only for a new level of wholesome, invigorating, health-sustaining foods and beverages, but also for those other items commonly purchased at the same time. You'll learn about the best types of products to use for health and beauty needs and for household cleaning.

You'll be inspired to develop and maintain healthy habits in the sections on the essentials of eating and exercise, and you'll explore ways to enhance your energy, health and stamina in the "chi" chapter. You'll also explore various types of natural healing modalities, receive an introduction to the helping professionals who practice them, and learn how to flush toxins out of your body once and for all.

In the final sections this courageous author invites you into his kitchen. You can see exactly what he uses to prepare delicious, healthful, and satisfying meals and snacks. For anyone who wants to start eating cleaner, more wholesome food that is kind to the consumer and the environment, this book is a must. Read it carefully and use its amazing detail and point-blank clarity to guide you to a new level of fulfillment and enjoyment in your health and your life.

I have worked for years to help physicians, mental health professionals, nurses, dietitians, and parents understand the nutritional aspects of attention deficit hyperactivity disorder, autism, and related conditions. As a producer of landmark and controversial videos, audiotapes, CDs and books on this topic, I know the kind of guts it takes for Larry Cook to produce a book of this magnitude, frankness, and tell-it-like-it-is helpfulness. As a champion of using natural methods as a useful and valid component of addressing medical and psychiatric conditions, I wholeheartedly recommend this book to you.

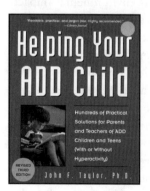

John F. Taylor, Ph.D.
Author,
Helping Your ADD Child
Nutrition & Neurochemistry: The ADD Link
and numerous other resources available from

www.ADD-Plus.com

Introduction
Change Your Lifestyle

In 1990 my life changed forever—and for the better—when I decided to adopt a strictly vegan vegetarian diet after reading *Diet For A New America* by John Robbins. A vegan (pronounced vee-gan) vegetarian doesn't eat anything that comes from animal sources, including meat, dairy, eggs and fish. Within months of adopting this lifestyle I lost 40 pounds, my health improved, my energy and stamina increased and I became a lot more pleasant to be around!

At the time, I thought that being vegetarian was enough to keep me healthy. Several years later, though, I discovered organic farming, macrobiotic eating, botanical body care, whole food supplements, natural medicine, holistic dentistry, non-toxic cleaning supplies, natural food stores, and so on, until I was firmly rooted in what is now termed "natural living." My interest in this lifestyle continued to climb, and by 1999 I had read dozens of books and scanned hundreds of Web sites on the topic. I applied what I learned to my daily living, with great success, and decided I wanted to share with others what I had discovered.

In June of 2000, while living in Bozeman, Montana, I was inspired to launch and publish a natural living magazine, even though I had no prior publishing experience. By August of 2002 I had successfully launched, published and sold two advertiser-supported magazines devoted to natural living—one in Montana, the other in Seattle. Over the course of those two years I distributed 16 issues with a combined circulation of over

250,000. Today, the Montana *Natural Life News & Directory*—with a current bi-monthly circulation of 12,000—continues to thrive and grow under new ownership. Unfortunately, the Seattle-based *EcoVision Journal* folded after I sold it.

Meanwhile, I have turned my attention toward putting my knowledge and experience into this book, which is the result of thousands of hours of research and practical application, as well as feedback from friends, clients, magazine readers, and professionals from diverse fields within the natural/holistic lifestyle community.

Natural Living Principles

The principles of natural living are based on the belief that there is a divine intelligence behind the operation of the body, as well as all of life. When given the *right conditions*, divine intelligence heals, rejuvenates and facilitates vibrant health. Conversely, when given the *wrong conditions*, divine intelligence is unable to operate properly, and sickness and disease can take hold. This book is about understanding both the *right* and *wrong conditions* that can lead to vibrant health or degenerative disease.

There is perhaps no greater way to understand divine intelligence than to observe the workings of nature, which is where the word "natural" in natural living comes from. Accordingly, natural living lifestyle adherents consciously choose to use products and services that are as close to nature as possible (e.g., in their *original* state), including food, remedies and philosophies; and they avoid products, services and philosophies that are not in harmony with nature (e.g., poisonous or slightly toxic substances found in most of today's food, beauty and cleaning products, conventional cleaners, etc.).

Each chapter in this book focuses on a specific topic that will help you join the growing number of people living (and loving!) a natural lifestyle.

Lifestyle Choices for Health

There is a philosophy to the natural living lifestyle: we have the power to create either *right* or *wrong conditions* for the divine intelligence flowing through us. The *goal* is to make *choices* that encourage the *right conditions* and diminish the *wrong conditions*. Based on my research and personal application of these principles, here is an outline of the *right conditions*, which are the foundation of this book:

1) Don't consistently pollute the body with minute amounts of toxins.
   • Chapters 1 and 2
2) Detoxify the body of chemical toxins and biological pathogens.
   • Chapters 7 and 8
3) Feed the body the highest quality nutrient-dense food available.
   • Chapters 1, 2, 3, 4, 5 and the Appendix
4) Choose plant-based (botanical) body care and household products for their safety and effectiveness.
   • Chapter 4
5) Use nutrient-dense supplements to ensure maximum nutrition.
   • Chapter 6
6) Exercise for energy, weight loss, confidence and detoxification.
   • Chapter 8
7) Build the "life force energy" in the body for maximum endurance, poise and power. (In Oriental medicine this life force energy is known as "chi." It runs through all living things, and its unblocked flow through the body ensures optimal health.)
   • Chapter 9
8) Utilize holistic dentistry, holistic medicine and holistic remedies to address the root cause of health issues and to support and facilitate the body's innate ability to heal itself. Question toxic medicine, which manages symptoms with drugs or surgery, sometimes suppressing natural bodily functions, and prolonging problems indefinitely.
   • Chapters 10 and 11
9) Continue to learn, and apply, the teachings of experts in the field of natural living.
   • Chapter 4 and Resources
10) Apply these principles simultaneously for a comprehensive multi-dimensional upgrading of your health or remedying of problems.

There are a wide variety of resources available that teach certain aspects of natural living. While most of them delve into a narrow range of specific topics, I have chosen to give you an overview of the essentials of multiple topics. I want you to get the "big picture" so you can quickly embark on the natural living lifestyle. This book will bring you up to speed on most of the issues so you can intelligently choose the best course of action for yourself and your family. Once you have this overview and embark on the natural living lifestyle path, consider gaining more in-depth knowledge about these topics by reading the selected resources I highlight and hyperlink throughout the book (this book is available in both print and e-book formats), or read some of the many sources of information found in the Resources section.

Mainstream Media, Government Agencies and Big Business

By the time you finish reading this book, I suspect you will see that big profits, inordinate power and systemic corruption can cloud the judg-ment of many who set governmental policies, practice medicine, report on health-related issues or develop and sell products. Most of what you will read in this book is not reported in the mainstream media because the mainstream media is owned and controlled by its advertisers: phar-maceutical giants, multi-national biotech food companies, chemical pro-ducers, medical conglomerates and the like. The media follows the lead of their advertisers, otherwise advertising dollars would be yanked and the media empires would collapse.

Governmental agencies such as the FDA and the USDA are very heavily influenced by the well-financed multinational corporations who have a vested interest in their profitable products, even if they are not good for us. Governmental agencies don't always provide their intended protection and can be hoodwinked into allowing harmful products onto the market. Worse still, truly helpful, safe and effective natural therapies are often locked into legal constraints that make it difficult, *or illegal,* for us to obtain them. I discuss this at length in Chapter 10. [For an excellent discourse on how natural remedies have been and are being deliberately suppressed, read John Robbin's *Reclaiming Our Health.*]

Sadly, this brings us to the allopathic medical establishment, which makes more money by keeping us slightly sick (with drug management) than from following effective natural cures. The use and discussion of natu-ral medicine is heavily discouraged and even mocked among their ranks, as you'll soon discover. *[In reference to allopathic medicine, I'm referring only to the standard treatments of degenerative disease, not for the acute care of trauma-induced injuries from accidents or corrective surgery due to birth defects and such,* as allopathic medicine is quite helpful in these circumstances.]

Your best protection is education, and I don't mean from your family M.D., TV nightly news, the daily newspaper or weekly magazines. Rather, check out my Resources and Bibliography for Web sites and books I highly recommend. John Robbins is one of my favorite authors in this regard, and there are plenty of other writers and sources offering sound, practical and well-researched advice for the natural living lifestyle. The book section of any natural foods store is a great place to continue your education in these matters.

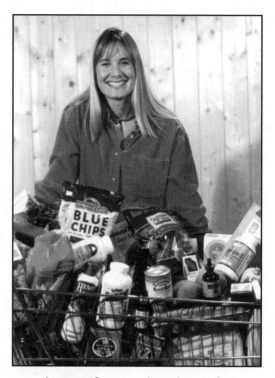

Shopping for natural products is fun!

Finally, living a natural lifestyle is easier than you think, and very rewarding. Everything discussed in this book is easy to do, once you form the habit. In the Conclusion I put everything together for you so you can quickly and easily begin the natural living lifestyle—for better health, happiness and prosperity!

1
Water
Make it Pure

The water you drink, cook with, bathe in or wash your clothes and dishes with may contain arsenic, lead, copper and other heavy metals. It might also contain fertilizer residues, asbestos, cyanides, herbicides and pesticides that have leached into groundwater from the soil or have been carried through plumbing pipes. There are about 30,000 hazardous waste sites and 16,000 landfills (along with thousands of illegal dumping sites) that contaminate groundwater. Several hundred thousand underground storage tanks in this country are thought to be leaking paints, solvents, toxic chemicals and petroleum products. Sewer surface runoff and rainwater from oil-slicked or salt-treated highways are additional sources of water pollution. Biological pathogens are another source of impurity: viruses, bacteria and parasites may lurk in your water.

We can be thankful that our obsession with chlorination has eliminated cholera and typhoid. While we don't have the overt problems faced by Third World countries, cities across the U.S. are now admitting that municipal water supplies are not as clean and safe as was previously believed. The Natural Resources Defense Council reports there are approximately 900,000 illnesses and 100 deaths per year due to contaminated water,[1] while the Centers for Disease Control report 900 deaths from water-borne illnesses each year. Best-selling health author Ann Louise Gittleman (*How To Stay Young and Healthy in a Toxic World*), citing statements from both *USA Today* and the *New York Times* in 1995, says that one in five of us drink water contaminated with feces, radiation or parasites. Those of us living in homes built before June 1988 (when lead pipes were banned for use in plumbing systems) may be drinking contaminated water because of lead leaching through our water pipes.

According to a special report by *Organic Style* magazine—based on a survey of 712 utilities around the country—arsenic poisoning is widespread.[2] The survey also revealed an unfortunate irony: in 1979, oil companies started adding methyl tertiary butyl ether (MTBE) to gasoline in order to make it burn more cleanly and reduce air pollution, yet MTBE has contaminated water supplies across the nation and can remain in groundwater for years. It leaks from underground storage tanks at gas stations, quickly spreading through underground water reserves and wells.

Approximately 25 percent of U.S. homes have septic systems, which may contaminate groundwater with fecal bacteria. If you draw water from a well or live on or near a ranch or farm, chemical residues may have leached into the water from fertilizers, pesticides and animal excrement. Nitrates are of particular concern in farm wells; ingesting these toxins creates free radicals that contribute to nutritional deficiencies and degenerative diseases.[3] Parasites such as giardia and cryptosporidium pose an additional risk.

Though polluted water isn't often detectable by sight, smell or taste, signs of polluted water include cloudiness, murkiness, foaming, or an odd smell or taste. Utility companies send yearly *Consumer Confidence* reports to homeowners each July; if you miss it (or are a renter) call the EPA's Safe Drinking Water Hotline (800-426-4791) and ask for a copy of your utility's report. You can also have your tap water tested by your state lab. To locate one, go to www.epa.gov and search "state certification officer" or call National Testing Laboratories, Ltd. at 800-458-3330. Another option is to contact the Environmental Working Group's Web site (www.ewg.org). Follow the link to "tap water" and then to "In the Drink," a database with information on water sources throughout America. Search for your community to determine the assessed health of your neighborhood water.

Livestock Industry—Mega-Users and Mega-Polluters

Though general industry uses or pollutes an almost incomprehensible amount of water, the livestock industry is undoubtedly the great water hog. *Meat production uses more water than the rest of the nation combined.*[4] For example, according to the research of John Robbin's, author of *Diet For A New America*, it takes 25 gallons of water to produce a pound of wheat, yet 2,500 gallons of water to produce a pound of beef. Besides irrigating land used to grow feed and fodder for livestock, enormous quantities of water are needed to wash away their excrement. While it used to be reintroduced to the soil as natural fertilizer, modern practices predominantly use synthetic fertilizers, thus leaving 130 *times* more excrement than humans produce—untreated—to drain into our water supply!

Chlorine Treatment

With so many pollutants soaking into groundwater and flowing through municipal pipes, it's no wonder our cities look for inexpensive, effective ways to clean it up. While some cities don't treat water at all and others filter it, most add chemicals to kill bacteria. The EPA considers "bacteriologically safe" water to be "pure," and recommends that tap water have a pH between 6.5 and 8.5. Chlorine is the highly toxic chemical most commonly used to "purify" city water.

Chlorine does destroy pathogenic bacteria; unfortunately, it isn't "target-specific" and also destroys our friendly intestinal bacteria required for proper digestion and a strong immune system. Chlorine has been linked to cardiovascular disease and cancer,[5] and it isn't effective against cryptosporidium, an increasingly virile parasite. Since chlorine will evaporate after it comes out of the tap, many people let water stand for half an hour or so to improve taste. However, chlorine combines with organic substances in the water to form chloroform, a cancer-causing chemical that does *not* evaporate.

Fluoridation

Part of the controversy over fluoride is due to confusion over calcium fluoride, used in the original tooth decay-prevention tests, and sodium fluoride, a highly toxic industrial waste product from the phosphate fertilizer industry. Unfortunately, it's sodium fluoride that's added to city water supplies. Many municipal water districts contain fluoride levels much higher than one part per million, originally set as the acceptable limit by the EPA.[6] Sodium fluoride kills most of our beneficial enzymes, attacks the hypothalamus gland (considered the master gland of the endocrine

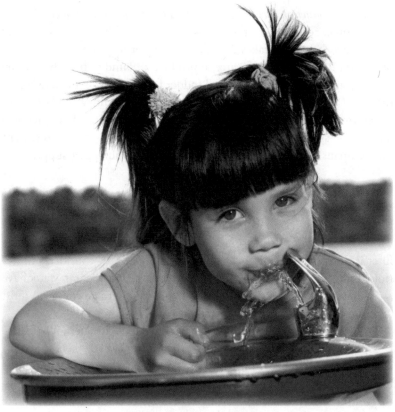

Fluoridated water puts our children at risk.

system), inhibits proper functioning of the thyroid gland (responsible for metabolism), can cause weakening of the bones (called skeletal fluorosis) and can cause dental fluorosis in children.[7] Dental fluorosis, a mineralization disorder of the teeth that degrades the enamel, is an irreversible condition caused by excessive ingestion of fluoride during the tooth forming years. In fact, contrary to the propaganda we hear in the media, the largest survey ever done on tooth decay—conducted by the *National Institute of Dental Research*—found *no* difference in tooth decay between fluoridated and non fluoridated communities in the U.S., when measured in terms of DMFT (Decayed, Missing & Filled Teeth).[8]

Sodium fluoride is also a very powerful central nervous system toxin that can adversely affect human brain functioning and diminish IQ, even at low doses.[9] Since over-ingestion of fluoride impairs the thyroid gland,[10] it probably contributes to the alarming rate of obesity in the U.S. In short, sodium fluoride—an industrial waste product added to most of our water supply—is an insidious poison that we should completely avoid.

Former *Christian Science Monitor* reporter Christopher Bryson's book, *The Fluoride Deception,* describes in detail the part fluoride played during the development of the atomic bomb, subsequent cover-ups and the foisting of this substance on the American public. While approximately 67 percent of American cities fluoridate municipal water, Europe has almost unanimously rejected it—only 2 percent of the entire continent allows water fluoridation. Over 80 U.S. cities have rejected fluoride since 1996. For more information on the dangers of fluoride, visit the Fluoride Action Network's website at www.fluoridealert.org.

If you're opposed to municipal water fluoridation, contact your City Council, county health board and state legislators—your efforts can make a difference! In Washington State, a group of citizens, cities and private water companies challenged the fluoride mandate in Pierce County, arguing that the health board had overreached its power: that the fluoridation order amounted to an illegal tax, and that it would force unwanted medical treatment on citizens. In May 2004, the Washington State Supreme Court ruled that a health board can not order all water systems within its jurisdiction to fluoridate.

Alternative Water Treatment: Ozone

While many argue that we need chlorine to keep our drinking water safe and that we can't afford other sanitation systems, much of Western Europe uses ozone gas and ultraviolet light to purify municipal water supplies. Since passage of The Safe Drinking Water Act Amendments in 1986, a number of cities in the U.S. have shown interest in ozone treatment. As of 1998, there were 264 water plants using this method. Mitsubishi Electric has developed commercial ozone water treatment technologies that are environmentally friendly. When combined with activated carbon filtration, ozonation removes agricultural chemicals and high-tech industrial wastes. Ozone is not only the strongest disinfectant known for potable water treatment, but it is also extremely versatile: it can enhance taste, remove undesirable color, destroy harmful algae and oxidize many organic compounds.

While it's not simple, ozone treatment has been shown to be economically viable both for large (commercial) and small (communities of less than 10,000 people) water treatment systems. In some cases it's actually cheaper than a chlorination/aeration system.[11] Clearly, ozonation is a viable alternative for municipal water supplies, and is worth serious consideration.

Bottled Water

As bottled water has become more popular, it has also come under scrutiny. Most states have no rules governing labeling; unfortunately, unscrupulous companies use misleading advertising, actually selling tap water as "natural spring water" or the like. While most companies are probably above board, nearly all package their product in plastic, a problem in its own right. Most plastic leaches into the water, particularly when transported in hot weather, sitting for days in metal trucks. Mountain Valley is a reputable company aware of this issue.

Larger containers are available in polycarbonate—a glass-like, non-porous plastic that doesn't leach plastics or dioxins (check out www.new-waveenviro.com or www.plasticsinfo.org) that can be filled with filtered water, dispensed at your local natural food store. These containers are slightly blue in color and are usually available in pint, 1/2 gallon, one, three or five gallon sizes. Alternatively, you can buy a three to five gallon glass jug that can be used with a ceramic pot reservoir. Clean the reservoir, jug and spigot monthly by running a 50/50 mixture of hydrogen peroxide and baking soda, then rinse with at least four gallons of tap water before filling it again.

Water Filters for the Home

Since most municipalities offer less than ideal water out of your tap, and driving to the store every few days for bottled water can be cumbersome, I suggest you install a high-quality filter that will not only remove heavy metals, pathogens and other contaminants, but will also remove chlorine, and *especially* fluoride. Ideally, you can install a full service filter for drinking, cooking, bathing and laundry. If not, then at least consider a filter for your drinking water and for your shower.

Best-selling health and beauty author Kat James (*The Truth About Beauty*) suggests a shower filter for screening chlorine from your skin and hair. "Most people are unaware of the ways that chlorinated shower water can undermine their efforts at beautiful skin, hair and health," she writes. Chlorine causes a cumulative burden to the skin, compromising its protective acid mantle barrier and causing oxidative damage. She suggests a shower filter utilizing the newer zinc-copper filter technology[12] that works with heat much better than carbon filters do.

There is a difference between water purification and water filtration. Purification refers to water that is as close to pure H_2O as possible, and is actually a government specified standard. Distilled water meets this standard and is considered by some to be an excellent choice for drinking, while others find it has serious drawbacks (see discussion below). Filtration removes most "suspended" material, leaving minerals and other potentially toxic water-soluble substances in the water. There are absorbent filters (usually carbon), micro filtration systems that run water through tiny pores, and ion-exchange resin filters. No filter will remove all contaminants, as each pore of even the finest filter is large enough for some viruses to permeate. Nature gives us a perfect example of water filtration: as water cascades through streams, and as it seeps through the soil and rocks to the water table, bacteria leeching into the rocks are replaced with minerals. Let's look at various ways to recreate the effectiveness of nature's method.

Reverse Osmosis

Reverse osmosis (RO) is effective in removing bacteria, viruses and parasites. Some of the more modern units take out nearly all toxins, gases and minerals. Water is pre-filtered to remove suspended matter and dissolve solids, then forced through a very fine semi-permeable membrane, which separates pure water molecules from remaining contaminants. The purified water is stored in a pressurized tank. When "tapped," it passes through an activated carbon post filter, ensuring the best possible taste.

RO water acts as a chelating agent—like a magnet, it draws out and flushes toxins. Since it pulls out important minerals along with impurities, it's important to take an ionic trace mineral supplement[13] if you choose this method. Another disadvantage of reverse osmosis is that it discharges about three gallons of wastewater for every purified gallon.

Distilled Water

This is the water used in many scientific labs. The process involves boiling water to a vapor. As the steam rises, it leaves behind most pollutants. The steam then goes into a condensing chamber, where it cools, condensing into purified water. Municipal water, however, often contains hydrocarbons, which have a lower boiling point than water. If you're purifying city water, be sure your distillation system has a "fractional" valve system that lets off the hydrocarbon gases, or a final-stage charcoal filter.

There is differing opinion among health proponents regarding distilled water. It leaches inorganic minerals rejected by cells and tissues out of the body—a good thing, according to James Balch, M.D., co-author of *Prescription for Nutritional Healing.* He believes it's the only water to drink, suggesting it be supplemented with two tablespoons of mineral drops for every five gallons of water to replace trace minerals. On the other hand, Ann Louise Gittleman points out that distillation can vaporize and concentrate chloroform and other chemicals, and removes essential trace minerals. She advises against its regular use, and suggests that if you do buy distilled water you look for "double distilled," a process not done by most companies.

Paul Pitchford, author of *Healing With Whole Foods,* recommends that water treated with either reverse osmosis or distillation be left in an open glass container for at least a day, and exposed to sunlight whenever possible.

Carbon, Activated Charcoal and Ceramic Filters

Unlike reverse osmosis and distillation, activated charcoal filtered water retains water-soluble minerals. If you don't have nitrate, nitrites or sodium fluoride in your water and the filter is renewed or replaced when its capacity is exhausted, this option can be a good way to go. Since these filters are less expensive than RO filters or distillers, they may be a necessary option even if you do have sodium fluoride. If so, you can stir a teaspoon of calcium powder (Dr. Bronner's Calcium-Magnesium Powder works well) into each gallon of filtered water. The fluoride combines with the calcium to form calcium fluoride, believed to be harmless in small doses. Let it settle to the bottom of the container and use the water off the top.

Health advocate and author Ann Louise Gittleman recommends ceramic filtration, since the ceramic is "bacteriostatic," preventing the formation of bacteria. This method has been used around the world for over 140 years and is a great way to eliminate parasites. Gittleman recommends the Doulton Ceramic Filter, made of ultra-fine ceramic with pores that trap particles as small as 0.5 microns. In a three-stage process, the pores first remove contaminants. Next, a carbon core eliminates dirt, odor, chlorine, pesticides and other pollutants. A heavy metal compound removes lead and copper. An ultraviolet light unit can be installed on the kitchen faucet or under the sink for added protection against bacteria and viruses.

Water Filters: My Suggestion

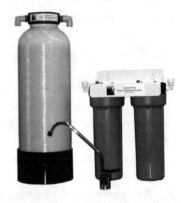

I've researched water filtration systems, and I'd like to give you my personal suggestion. Custom Pure *MB Filter Series* (www.custompure.com) offers deionization resin filtration—a filtration technique used by the electronics and biomedical industries to obtain ultra pure water—along with activated carbon absorption. This combination produces distilled quality, delicious tasting water and removes chlorine and chloroform, fluoride, lead, arsenic, asbestos, rust, copper, sodium, sulfates, nitrates, sediments, giardia, cryptosporidium and other dissolved solids and volatile organic chemicals. The system includes an optional ultraviolet sterilizer and a ceramic cartridge. If your water is microbiologically contaminated, these optional features are required in order to achieve desired results. The company offers a limited lifetime warranty and free water testing for monitoring filter performance.[14] Their online questionnaire, *Choosing a Drinking Water System,* is very helpful in determining your needs. I've been using a Custom Pure water filter for the last three years.

Water Softeners

Depending on where you live, your tap water can be classified as either relatively "hard" or "soft." Hard water contains much more calcium than does soft water, which contains more magnesium. Soft water saves on gas and electric bills, because it takes nearly 30 percent more gas to produce hot water from hard water. If you have an electric hot water heater, you'll use between 21 and 68 percent more energy with hard water than with soft. Softening the water removes large-molecule pollutants like lead and arsenic. Traditional softeners add sodium to the water, making it a poor choice for drinking and a burden to our soils. Fortunately, new technologies employ magnetic water conditioners that retain the beneficial minerals found in "hard" water as well as introduce cleansing benefits associated with "soft" water. GMX International (http://clearwatermax.com/home.htm), based in Chico, California, offers a university-tested magnetic water conditioning system that uses a salt-free solution effective for both commercial and residential use.

Our Water—the Big Picture

Ecologists report that the areas around rivers, lakes and streams have borne the heaviest burden from human use. Biologists tell us that aquatic species are disappearing at a faster rate than terrestrial ones. Consider the following statistics, compiled by the Living Waters Project:[15]

- Since the 1800s the lower 48 states have lost just over half their wetlands
- Approximately 40 percent of rivers, lakes and coastal water in the U.S. don't meet basic safety standards for drinking and swimming
- In the U.S, 35 percent of both freshwater fish and amphibians, and 57 percent of fresh-water mussels, are at risk.

The Colorado River doesn't always reach the ocean anymore—it's dried up from being over-utilized for lawn-watering and other uses in the Southwest. Many rivers and water sources in the East face the same situation. Clearly, water is becoming a precious commodity, and corporations are poised to globalize and negotiate it on the market, rather than conserve it as a resource available to everyone. Water is becoming the oil of the 21st century. The film *Thirst* (www.thirstthemovie.com) examines water conflicts on three continents and shows that popular opposition to the privatization of *our* water sparks remarkable coalitions.

All of us are responsible for our priceless, dwindling resource: water. As the ancients knew, it's the stuff of life—don't take it for granted. And remember to filter it before drinking!

2
Food
Avoid Synthetic

One of the greatest threats to the human race is the all-pervasive, on-going, deliberate manipulation of our food supply—from the farm to the shelf, and at every step in-between. Without a doubt, the contamination of our food with synthetic chemicals (e.g., pesticides, herbicides, heavy metals, preservatives, food dyes, stabilizers, artificial flavorings, fake vitamins, growth hormones, tranquilizers, antibiotics, etc., etc., ad nauseam) combined with production techniques that utterly decimate the intrinsic nutritional value of raw food (e.g., genetic engineering, irradiation, high-temperature processing, hydrogenation, etc.), is the primary root cause of degenerative disease in America and abroad.*

Our bodies are not designed to operate on nutritionally stripped, chemically laden food day in and day out. Daily intake of micro doses of toxins over the course of years or decades, and deprivation of optimum nutrition—which is contrary to what nature intends—will certainly cause a degenerative disease to set in sooner or later.

To be free of degenerative disease, then, means we must abstain, as often as possible, from eating synthetic (man-derived) food. In this chapter I give an in-depth explanation of how most of our food is being deliberately compromised. For optimum health, avoid these foods, and instead embrace the foods I discuss in Chapter 3.

*Health and beauty aids are also loaded with synthetic chemicals, and most cleaning products use highly toxic chemicals, all of which can contribute to the decline of health.

Pesticides and Herbicides

"Pesticides are not 'safe.' They are produced
specifically because they are toxic to something."[1]
-U.S. EPA, Citizen's Guide to Pesticides, 1987

Chemical pesticides and herbicides are widely accepted in conventional farming as an indispensable tool to kill bugs and weeds that would otherwise infest growing crops. Yet there are other ways to control pests that don't dump toxins into the food supply, soil and groundwater. You wouldn't spray Raid* on your carrots or green beans, so why eat foods sprayed with insecticide? Pesticides, herbicides and fungicides accumulate in body cells, fatty tissue and in the nervous system. We can probably handle ingesting them once in a while, but these kinds of chemicals build up over time in our bodies and lead to disease.

Healthy soil, containing live worms, vigorous bacteria and other bio-activity,[2] makes plants resilient to infestations. Soil from farms that use synthetic chemical pesticides and fertilizers don't show these characteristics.

The information available on the harmful effects of synthetic chemical pesticides and herbicides is staggering. Unfortunately, this information is not widely disseminated and never reaches most people, so it's up to each of us to educate ourselves. Take a look at these facts:

- More than 1,000 new chemicals are introduced every year, the vast majority of which have not been adequately tested for human safety.[3]
- More than 4.7 billion pounds of poisonous pesticides and herbicides are sprayed on our food crops every year.[4]
- Each year, American farmers use more than forty million *tons* of synthetic chemical fertilizers on croplands.[5] Agrichemicals, including pesticides and herbicides, accumulate in our fat and weaken our immune systems by suppressing the function of white blood cells—the T helper and B cells that produce antibodies.[6]
- In 1996, global sales of pesticides topped 30 billion dollars.[7]

In 1962, Rachel Carson's book *Silent Spring* exposed the devastating effects of chemicals in our food and environment. The public outcry

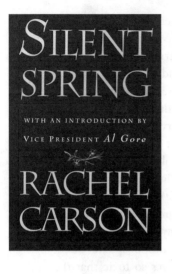

SILENT
SPRING

WITH AN INTRODUCTION BY

VICE PRESIDENT *Al Gore*

RACHEL
CARSON

that followed forced the banning of the lethal pesticide DDT[8] and changed the laws affecting our land, water and air.

At the time, the world-famous Mayo Clinic admitted hundreds of patients who had severe diseases of the blood organs, such as leukemia. Carson quoted Dr. Malcolm Hargraves in writing, "The vast majority of patients suffering from the blood dyscrasais and lymphoid diseases have a significant history of exposure to various hydrocarbons, which includes most of the pesticides of today. A careful medical history will almost invariably establish such a relationship." In fact, his team found that almost without exception these patients had a history of exposure to chemicals and sprays containing DDT, chlordane, benzene, lindane and petroleum distillates.[9]

Today, it's actually much worse. Remember Agent Orange, the toxic spray used by our military in Vietnam to destroy forests, which caused all kinds of health problems for our veterans and birth defects in their children? Two of the toxic chemicals found in Agent Orange, 2,4-D and 2,4,5-T, are sprayed on land used to grow feed for livestock.[10] 2,4,5-T contains dioxin, one of the most toxic chemicals in the world (far more toxic than DDT.)

Dioxin causes cancer, birth defects, miscarriages and death in lab animals at even *one part per trillion* and kills the animal almost immediately. The Environmental Protection Agency's Dr. Dianne Courtney called dioxin "by far the most toxic chemical known to mankind."[11] *Yet dioxin is legally used on the food we eat.*

Children are at very great risk. Here's some information from the Environmental Working Group:

> "Ten years after Alar [a pesticide for apples featured on *60 Minutes* that ultimately led to its being banned], apples still need a cleanup. An apple a day exposes your child to more than 30 pesticides over a year. [That's]

an average of four [pesticides] per apple, with six or eight not uncommon. In 1996, the most recent year the USDA tested apple samples, government labs detected a total of 39 different pesticide residues on 530 samples. Ninety-eight percent (98%) of the apple samples tested were positive for pesticide residues. Pesticides…can damage the human brain and nervous system, disrupt hormones, and cause cancer.

More than a million preschoolers consume at least 15 pesticides a day in food, according to our latest study of government data. Some 324,000 kids age five and under exceed federal safety standards every day for just one neurotoxic[12] insecticide, methyl parathion. Methyl parathion is the most toxic organophosphate insecticide approved for use on food. It's so toxic that the EPA's 'daily' safe dose for the compound is 0.000025 milligrams per kilogram of human body weight. A 154-pound person would exceed the EPA daily dose by eating less than two one-millionths of a gram of the chemical (.002 milligrams). Some apples and peaches are so contaminated with methyl parathion that a kid can exceed the government's safe daily limits with just two bites. A 154-pound adult eating such an apple would ingest only half of the current safe daily dose, whereas it would put a 44-pound child 67 percent over his or her 'safe' limit."[13]

Organophosphate pesticides inhibit the enzyme acetylcholinesterase, a key molecule required to permit the regeneration of acetylcholine at neuromuscular junctions and thereby control nerve to muscle transmission. Many organophosphorus compounds damage nerves directly, creating adverse conditions that are largely irreversible. Animal studies show that organophosphorus compounds damage the central nervous system. Neurological poisoning may take months or years to show up. Concentrated organophosphorus compounds are used to produce nerve gas, and a few drops are quickly lethal.[14] Symptoms of poisoning include stomach and intestinal cramps, vomiting, diarrhea and 'pinpoint' pupils. These pesticides change chemically as they age, becoming even more toxic. Philip J. Landrigna, pediatrician and chair of the National Academy of Sciences Committee, spoke about the risks of agrichemicals ingested by children. He said, "There should be a presumption of greater toxicity to infants and children. In such cases, the National Academy of Sciences panel called for exposure standards ten times more stringent than would normally be applied."[15]

Environmentalist and researcher Lewis Regenstein tells us in his book *How to Survive in America the Poisoned*, "Despite the overwhelming evidence that pesticides cause cancer and are extremely dangerous to humans and the environment, almost none of these chemicals has ever been 'banned' by the government in the true sense of the word."[16] Most chemicals that have been banned in the United States are shipped abroad to countries like Mexico, which ships its produce back to the U.S. laden with those same chemicals![17]

Two dozen pesticides and herbicides used today disrupt the human endocrine system.[18] In late 1995, a multidisciplinary group of international experts[19] gathered in Erice, Sicily for a work session on "Environmental Endocrine-Disrupting Chemicals: Neural, Endocrine and Behavioral Effects."[20] The committee wrote: "Thyroid hormones are essential for normal brain function throughout life. Interference with thyroid hormone function during development leads to abnormalities in brain and behavioral development. The eventual results of moderate to severe alterations of thyroid hormone concentrations, particularly during fetal life, are motor dysfunction of varying severity, including cerebral palsy, mental retardation, learning disability, attention deficit hyperactivity disorder, hydrocephalus, seizures and other permanent neurological abnormalities. Similarly, exposure to man-made chemicals during early development can impair motor function, spatial perception, learning, memory, auditory development, fine motor coordination, balance, and attention processes; in severe cases, mental retardation may result. Because certain PCBs and dioxins are known to impair normal thyroid function, we suspect that they *contribute to learning disabilities, including attention deficit hyperactivity disorder and other neurological abnormalities.*"[21] [italics mine]

While we all need to be concerned about foods doused with pesticides, herbicides and similar chemicals, farm workers are exposed to significantly higher risks. What happens to their health is a telltale sign. The December 1997 edition of Indian Express Newspaper tells the story:

> "In California's onion fields, farm workers, including children, are exposed to methyl parathion, a potent nerve toxin. Among Florida's strawberry fields they encounter captan, a probable human carcinogen. In Midwestern cucumber patches they face endosulfan, a chemical that may cause a host of health problems because of its similarity to human hormones. An unreleased US Department of Labor survey shows 123,000 children [between] the ages of 14 and 17 working in America's fields. There are thousands more under 14 who go uncounted. Children as young as four were found to be working in the fields and mothers who can't afford day care carry infants into the fields. In Ohio this summer, six-year-old Ramiro Silva and his sister picked pesticide-dusted cucumbers and ate them unwashed for lunch. Alejandra Renteria, also six, sometimes refused to wear rubber gloves[22] because they were too big and clumsy for her. 'My arms get itchy sometimes, but I like to work,' Renteria said. Itchy irritations are common in pesticide exposure."[23]

Farmers exposed to pesticides and herbicides often have elevated risks of leukemia, lymphoma, and other cancers. According to a 1997 study by the International Labor Organization, up to 14 percent of all occupational injuries in the agricultural sector and 10 percent of all fatal injuries can be attributed to pesticides.

About half of all illnesses reported in the state of California are associated with agricultural work, with approximately 1,000 cases of pesticide poisonings annually. Analysts believe this figure is low, estimating that up to 80 percent of all incidents may go unreported. Studies also show that pesticide chemicals interfere with hormones, disrupting the normal growth and development of mammals, birds, reptiles, amphibians and humans. Disturbing evidence includes reduced sperm counts in humans, nervous and immune system disorders in wildlife and humans, and increased birth defects and impaired sexual development in animals.

In 1977, 35 workers in a pesticide plant in Occidental, California were found to be sterile due to exposure to the pesticide DBCP. At least 2,000 more workers who applied the pesticide on banana plantations in Central America were also rendered sterile.[24] In 1978, California banned the pesticide and a year later the federal government banned all interstate use of DBCP. Nevertheless, DBCP manufacturers Dow Chemical and Shell Oil continue to sell it overseas.[25]

Research clearly shows the link between pesticides, herbicides and most diseases and cancers.[26] Why isn't this information broadcast by the media or the government or even discussed at universities? The answer, of course, has to do with money.

There are currently eight major players in the pesticide industry: Dow Chemical, Du Pont, Monsanto, Imperial Chemical Industries, Novartis, Rhone Poulenc, Bayer and Hoechst. These companies produce pharmaceuticals along with toxic pesticides, genetically modified seeds and industrial chemicals.[27] These same companies fund political campaigns and universities and spend millions on advertising. From 1979 to 1995, twelve of the leading chemical companies contributed more than seven million dollars to congressional campaigns. From 1979 to 1994, Monsanto and Dow gave $42.5 million to foundations and universities for pesticide research. Results are quite interesting: from 1989 to 1993, 74 percent of 43 studies on four chemicals funded by industry or corporations indicated that the chemical was safe. In contrast, only 27 percent of 118 studies funded by non-industry scientists showed favorable results. In California, only *2.6 percent* of the state Department of Pesticide Regulation (DPR) budget is allocated to research alternatives to pesticides.[28]

These large corporations also have a major influence on the media by funding newspaper and magazine articles, radio shows and television programs. The media may report on alternative solutions, but always consult experts funded by the chemical giants who ultimately *dismiss* alternative solutions.

The best way to avoid pesticides and herbicides in our food supply is to buy organically grown food. This topic is discussed in more detail in Chapter 3.

Genetically Modified Organisms

If you shop at a conventional supermarket, you may be putting more than you think into your cart. Between 60 to 70 percent[1] of the food you buy probably contains genetically modified organisms (GMOs). Since foods containing these organisms are not required to be labeled as such, fastidious label-readers may see a list of "nos" (no sugar, no additives, no preservatives…) and unwittingly toss something into the cart that contains "blind" GMO. Few foods are exempt: taco shells, tortilla chips, drink mixes, fish, corn syrup, products containing corn or soy, many vegetables—including eggplant, squash, tomatoes, corn, cabbage, lettuce, potatoes—even "veggie" burgers and baby formulas have been modified. Though agribusiness would have us believe we're buying bigger, better products, the facts show we should be very wary.

Viruses Spliced Into Food

Genetic modification involves altering the natural structure of DNA coding, often by bringing foreign DNA from another living thing to the target plant through a "vector," or carrier. Viruses are commonly used as vectors in genetic engineering, since they usually attack the host's cells and merge easily into its DNA. It's cutting and pasting at the submicroscopic level and, since this is difficult to keep track of, scientists often mark the vectors with antibiotic-resistant genes. Cells are then doused with antibiotics and those without the resistance (e.g., the natural cells) die. The use of antibiotic-resistant marker genes in food means that we consume those genes, more than likely causing the healthful bacteria in our bodies to become antibiotic-resistant as well.

Farmeceuticals and the New Pharmers

For centuries, farmers have saved seeds to replant for their next crop, or have used hybrid experimentation to create new varieties of plants, relying on nature to sanction the experiment. Today, however, many farmers are held economically hostage by a handful of giant corporations (say "Monsanto," spell D-U-P-O-N-T) who have placed patents on their genetically modified food plants, giving them exclusive control over that food and its seeds. Monsanto sells farmers genetically engineered seeds that are "Roundup Ready," often requiring them to sign a contract promising to use only those seeds and the corresponding Roundup herbicide, manufactured by Monsanto. Roundup is designed to kill virtually everything green in the field except the genetically engineered plant.

Some plants are genetically altered and reprogrammed to kill their own seeds. Referred to as "terminator technology," such seeds cannot be saved and replanted, which forces farmers to purchase new seeds each year from the manufacturer. Created by the U.S. Department of Agriculture (USDA) and Delta and Pine Land (a company owned by Monsanto), the technology was granted a patent so broad it allows terminator seeds to be used in the plants and seeds of all crops. Due to public outcry (over 7,000 people have written to the USDA expressing their opposition to its use), Monsanto pledged in late 1999 not to use it. There are, however, 27 similar patent holders who may or may not follow suit.

More Corporate Control

In their book, *Genetically Engineered Food: Changing the Nature of Nature*, Martin Teitel, Ph.D. and Kimberly Wilson note that, "Entire varieties of plants are now patented corporate products. In some cases, entire species are owned. Furthermore, this new technology is global, changing local ecology and tastes to a planetary monoculture enforced by intricate trade agreements and laws."

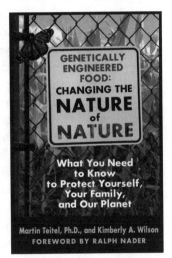

A Threat to Biodiveristy

Normally the boundaries between species are set by nature, but because of self-serving economic pressures, that's changing. In the last 20 years, genetic splicing has replaced nature's role in creating hybrid crops. Plant species in the wild are less vulnerable to insects and diseases than GMO crops because they have a broad genetic base to work from, whereas technologically engineered hybrids create an ever-shrinking genetic pool and erode the natural biodiversity inherent in cross-pollination. Gene-spliced "super salmon" are engineered to grow at four times the rate of their naturally spawned counterparts. The 'GM' fish are thus available year-round, filling the tummies of eager consumers and lining the pockets of developers. While some are delighted to enjoy the feast, others agree with physicist Dr. John Hagelin, who states: "When genetic engineers disregard the reproductive boundaries set by natural law, they run the risk of destroying our genetic encyclopedia, compromising the richness of our natural biodiversity, and creating 'genetic soup.' What this means to the future of our ecosystem, no one knows."

Environmental Hazards
Agribusiness knows from public opinion polls that demand for genetically engineered foods is low and that demand for labeling is high. Yet as of 1998 there are 58 million acres[2] of "genfoods" grown in the United States (of approximately 70 million acres worldwide), and *two-thirds* of the products on supermarket shelves have genetically engineered ingredients, including 35 percent of all corn, 55 percent of all soybeans and nearly half of all cotton.[3] Are we unwitting guinea pigs in the largest experiment in human history? Many scientists think so. Some fear that GMOs will be spread by bird, insect or wind to non-GM crops, as well as to wilderness areas. Unlike other pollution, genetic contamination can neither be contained nor cleaned up.

While most GM crops are heavily herbicide or pesticide dependent, some actually create their own. Monsanto's New Leaf Superior potato is engineered to produce "Bt" (Bacillus thuringiensis, a naturally occurring soil bacterium) in each cell. *The potato itself has been registered as a pesticide with the U.S. Environmental Protection Agency.* Since labeling is not required, there is no way of knowing that the potato you pick up in the grocery is New Leaf or a regular spud. Should you care?

In early 1999, genetically engineered potatoes were tested on rats at Rowett Research Institute. After only ten days the animals suffered substantial health effects, including weakened immune systems and changes in the development of their hearts, livers, kidneys and brains. Research scientist Dr. Arpad Pusztai was fired after he publicly announced his findings and stated that he would not eat genetically modified foods. A commission convened by his former employers found his work "deficient." However, another panel of 20 independent scientists confirmed both his data and his findings.[4]

Rationale Rebuttal

Biotechnologists claim that genetic engineering is safe and environmentally friendly, that it will feed the world and reduce the use of herbicides and pesticides, and that GMO foods are just like natural foods. But the reality is that transgenic crops are heavily dependent on the use of chemical fertilizers and pesticides, and often require increased irrigation, depleting already precious water resources. We reap no obvious benefits; the genetically modified products don't look or taste better than non-GMs; they don't cost less or provide better nutrition. In fact, these novel foods are of questionable nutritional value and safety; genfood might be more aptly named, "frankenfood," since no one really knows what this ill-conceived creature will do once it's off and running.

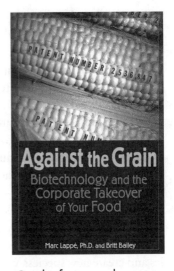

Against the Grain
Biotechnology and the Corporate Takeover of Your Food

Marc Lappé, Ph.D. and Britt Bailey

Get the facts on who wants to own our food supply.

Long-Term Health Effects?

Currently, there is no long-term safety testing of genetically modified organisms. Since genetic engineering can cause unexpected mutations in an organism, higher levels of toxicity in foods can be expected. Though extended shelf life may allow foods to appear fresh and luscious, the nutritional content of transgenic foods has been shown to be lower than that of foods grown traditionally. In 1999, the *Journal of Medicinal Food* published a study conducted by Dr. Marc Lappe; beneficial phytoestrogen compounds thought to protect against heart disease and cancer were found to be lower in genetically altered soybeans. Additionally, the antibiotically resistant genes within genfoods may be picked up by bacteria, which may infect us.[5] We might also expect increased pollution of food and water supplies, deletion of important food elements, decreased effectiveness of antibiotics, unforseen and undetected toxins, and sick or suffering livestock. A certain percentage of the population will more than likely have allergic reactions which, in some cases, may be severe.

Lobby for Labels

Without labels, public health agencies are powerless to trace problems that may occur. Codex, an agency of the UN World Health Organization, is an international group that sets food labeling standards. While it claims to have the public interest as its top priority, both the Canadian and U.S. delegations to Codex meetings have opposed the labeling of genetically modified food. Interestingly, in both countries nine or ten of thirteen and fourteen non-governmental positions, respectively, are filled by large corporations or industry groups. Some countries have chosen not to wait for Codex to wade through an eight-step process to create international food standards—British law currently requires that genetically modified foodstuffs be labeled.

Bioengineering is a very imprecise science. Unanswered questions seem worth pondering. Is it safe or even ethical to cross natural boundaries and create new species? What happens to the insects that feed on these transgenic crops? What happens when the wind carries the pollen from these plants to neighboring fields? What are the reproductive implications of altering the genetic structure of an animal? What effect will it have as these changes ripple through our intricate and profoundly interrelated ecosystem? If such questions concern you, consider shopping at a natural foods store to obtain organic food that has been certified as such, which is GMO-free. And contact The Campaign to Label Genetically Engineered Foods (www.thecampaign.org), the non-profit group spearheading action on changing laws regarding GMO food.

Irradiation

Eaten out lately? Chances are good that if you grabbed some fast food or ate at a corporate chain restaurant, part of your meal was irradiated. When sold in grocery stores, irradiated foods are supposed to be labeled, but restaurants, hospitals, schools and food services do not have to (and most times do not) notify their customers.

This so-called "purification" process exposes almost any food, especially meat, to gamma radiation in order to kill bacteria that can cause spoilage and/or food poisoning. The radiation may come from nuclear material such as cobalt 60 or cesium 137 (both highly toxic), from x-rays or electronic beams. Usually, 100,000 RADS is administered to meats, vegetables and fruits, and up to 3,000,000 RADS is administered to spices.[1] Supposedly, the food doesn't become radioactive, but other biochemical changes do occur—changes that have been shown to adversely affect both humans and animals.

Irradiation ionizes the atoms in food, knocking electrons out of orbit and creating free radicals, some of which recombine to form new, sometimes unknown compounds. Though stable, many of these compounds are toxic, such as formaldehyde, benzene, and lipid peroxides. Other free radicals cause destruction at the cellular level. Irradiated foods can lose up to 80 percent of their vitamins, especially vitamins A, C, E, K and B complex, as well as folic acid—the very substances needed to fight free radicals. Irradiation destroys the vital life force (chi energy), live enzymes (found in fresh foods and responsible for aiding both digestion and metabolic activity) and friendly bacteria needed to maintain health.

Animals fed irradiated foods have shown various results: tumors, kidney failure, reproductive problems, miscarriages and death of offspring. And those effects may not be limited to animals. In 1975, five malnourished children in India were fed irradiated wheat (at 75,000 RADS) for over three weeks. Four of the five children showed *gross chromosomal damage* just four weeks after initiation of the feeding, and the experiment was stopped. According to S.G. Srikantia, Professor of Food and Nutrition at the University of Mysore, India, such an increase in abnormalities strongly suggests a link to cancer.

Lost your appetite? You aren't alone. According to a 1997 CBS nationwide poll, 77 percent of the American public would not knowingly eat irradiated food. Recently, 98.2 percent of the Americans responding to the FDA's request for public comment said they wanted the current labeling law maintained or strengthened.[2] Labeling of irradiated food is not required if it is not packaged for resale to the public. The majority of Americans questioned about irradiation are against it, and say they want irradiated foods to be labeled as such. So the industry has come up with terms such as "electronic pasteurization," "pasteurization with x-rays" and "cold pasteurization." Whatever they call it, it's still irradiation.

Though its population clearly doesn't approve, the United States accepts irradiation for beef, pork, poultry, grains, vegetables, fruits, spices and teas. And if conventional agribusiness has its way, irradiation facilities containing highly toxic nuclear materials will be built around the country, increasing the risk of nuclear accidents such as the 1988 leak in Georgia, when radioactive cesium-137 water escaped from one facility, costing taxpayers $47 million to clean up. Internationally, there are over 150 irradiation facilities in over 40 countries. During a typical irradiation treatment, over 90 percent of both harmful and beneficial bacteria are destroyed. So, though E. coli is destroyed, so are the helpful bacteria that alert our noses with a foul smell once the food has gone bad. And, while the bacteria responsible for botulism are not killed, the natural enemies of botulism are destroyed during the irradiation process.

A hypothesis supported by many professionals is that E. coli and other harmful bacteria may become radiation resistant if irradiation becomes widespread. In fact, the Deinococcus radiodurans bacterium can survive 1.5 million RADS of gamma irradiation (that's 3,000 times the amount that would kill a person!) by reconstructing itself within 24 hours after being sliced to pieces by the radiation![3]

So, what's the underlying reason for all this nuking? Rampant fecal contamination of animals destined for slaughter appears to be the reason the meat industry is pushing so strongly for irradiation. Most food poisoning is caused by animal feces in food or water. Unsanitary and foul slaughterhouse conditions severely afflict that industry (read *Slaughterhouse: The Shocking Story of Greed, Neglect, and Inhumane Treatment Inside the U.S. Meat Industry*, by Gail Eisnitz). Rather than zapping the meat, wouldn't a better solution be to literally clean up their act?

Until then, we may want to consider eating little or no meat (hey, boycotting sends a mega-message to mega-business). And write your congressperson, or a supermarket/chain store CEO, as New Jersey Assemblyman John Kelly did. Kelly wrote to Wal-Mart CEO Lee Scott after learning of Wal-mart's plan to sell irradiated meat:

> "Contrary to what irradiation proponents would have you believe, the science supporting the safety of irradiated food is woefully lacking and borders on being nonexistent. It is a smoke and mirrors science at its best. In approving food irradiation, the FDA ignored the recommendations of its own toxicology committees. Rather than conduct toxicology studies that would address the issue of long-term health effects, the FDA

chose to approve irradiation based on, in their words, 'theoretical calculations in radiation chemistry.'

There is a body of research on the safety of irradiated food that raises concern, and yet is ignored by the FDA. One recurring theme is the effect of irradiated food on reproduction. A number of studies have raised the issue of miscarriages and fertility. USDA studies found that an irradiated diet resulted in 83 percent fewer offspring. I would hope you choose not to participate in this experiment with your customer's health and refrain from marketing what I refer to as 'birth control burgers.'"[4]

Now, where is the trusty FDA when we need it? On the wrong side, it would appear. From over 2,000 studies on food irradiation, they chose only *five* as cite-worthy, discarding or ignoring those which suggested that irradiation can cause harmful effects in animals or humans. The five studies accepted by the FDA have been strongly criticized because of their methodology and interpretation of data. For example, since irradiation is known to deplete vitamins, vitamin supplements were fed to the rats in one of the studies. In two more of the five studies, 55,000 RADS or less was administered to foods fed to the animals—significantly lower than the 100,000 RADS currently used to treat food for human consumption. In one of the studies, four litters of rats were still-born on the 200,000 rad diet, whereas only one such litter was still-born in the control group. In another study, five of sixteen dogs fed irradiated foods had birth defects.[5] Yet the FDA still approved irradiation based on the findings from these five studies!

For those who care to read it, there is enough scientific literature to suggest that eating irradiated food can cause health problems. In fact, in June of 1987, the House Committee on Energy and Commerce and the Subcommittee on Health and the Environment heard expert testimonies from four academic scholars;[6] all four spoke against irradiation. George Tritsch, Ph.D., stated, "I am opposed to consuming irradiated food because of the abundant and convincing evidence in the referenced scientific literature that the condensation products of the free radicals formed during irradiation produce statistically significant increases in carcinogenesis, mutagenesis and cardiovascular disease in animals and man."[7]

Richard Piccioni, Ph.D., states, "We feel that there is no assurance in the scientific literature or the arguments of the FDA that the widespread irradiation of food will not be a significant, if silent, threat to the public health."[8] Donald Louria, Ph.D., states, "I do not believe that irradiated foods have been shown to be safe for general consumption [and]…the effects of irradiation on the nutrient contents of food are not established."[9] S.G. Srikantia, B.Sc., B.B.S., D.Sc., states, "[The National Institute of Nutrition]…stands behind its statement that eating irradiated wheat-based diets is associated with undesirable consequences."[10] For an excellent source of compiled articles, books and news items related to the ill effects of irradiation, visit the Organic Consumers Association at www.organicconsumers.org and click on their "irradiation" link—you'll find plenty of facts and figures.

If you want to avoid irradiated food, buy organic and ask the restaurants you frequent if they know whether or not the food they serve has been irradiated.

Food Additives

"No additive shall be deemed safe if it is
found to induce cancer in humans or animals…"
The Delaney Clause—1958 Food Additives Amendment

As if it weren't enough that toxic pesticides, herbicides and fungicides are sprayed onto food crops, most manufacturers then lace what we eat with a cornucopia of harmful synthetic chemicals during processing, even though the Delaney Clause specifically forbids it.[1] Since 1959, more than 25 chemical food additives have been banned because they cause cancer or other serious diseases in laboratory animals. Dozens of other additives are currently under review by the U.S. Food and Drug Administration.[2] You might be familiar with some of these substances: food dyes, preservatives, flavorings, stabilizers, anti-mold agents, and so on. Unfortunately, our bodies can't use these chemicals; physiologically, we react to them as we would to a poison. Research has linked some synthetic additives with hyperactivity and behavioral changes—as well as with asthma (which frequently afflicts those with ADHD), cancer and other serious ailments.

Manufacturers use these chemicals because after food is harvested, it can spoil quickly.[3] So large multinational corporations, seeking to maximize profits and minimize losses during shipping and storage, alter fresh foods using a process that makes them last longer, but strips them of life force[4] and nutrition. Foods are suffused with synthetic flavorings (because the natural flavor was removed), preservatives (to keep what's left of the natural food from spoiling), synthetic food dyes (to ensure a uniform appearance at all times—while making food resemble what shoppers think the real thing would look like) and sometimes synthetic vitamins (to create the illusion of nutrition).

This is *not* what nature intended for us to eat! We become ill from all these chemicals—these toxins—circulating through and ultimately being stored in our bodies. Yet, despite the dangers that food additives pose to our health, their use is widespread. The average additive consumption per person, including pesticides, is about nine to ten pounds a year.[5] By the time an American child is five years old, he will have consumed more than 7.5 pounds of food additives through preservatives, emulsifiers, lubricants, bleaching agents, synthetic sweeteners, flavor enhancers and artificial colors and flavors.[6] In 1995, the worldwide flavors-and-fragrance market was worth $12 billion. Food flavorings account for 40 percent of this market ($5 billion) and represent approximately 14 percent of the total food-additive market.[7]

Eliminate Food Additives; Improve Behavior
The late Ben F. Feingold, M.D., author of *Why Your Child Is Hyperactive*, was among the first medical professionals to maintain that synthetic food dyes, preservatives and flavorings can cause severe behavioral changes in both children and adults. Feingold's research helped get some toxic synthetics banned in the United States. His pioneering work also led to the *Feingold Diet* for ADHD, which eliminates all foods containing synthetic dyes and food flavorings. Also eliminated are the synthetic antioxidant preservative chemicals butylated hydroxyanisole (BHA), butylated hydroxytoluene (BHT) and tertiary butylhydroquinone (TBHQ), as well as aspirin and other salicylates (naturally occurring compounds found in some fruits, vegetables and toiletries). Thousands of children who have followed this diet showed marked improvement in behavior—and often recovered from ADHD.[8]

Food additives and the health problems they can cause.*

Erythrosine FD&C Red No.3 (E 127 Europe)	Sequential vascular response Elevation of protein-bound iodide Thyroid tumors, Chromosomal damage
Citrus Red No.2 (used in dyeing orange peels)	Cancer in animals
Allura Red AC, FD&C Red No.40	Tumors (e.g., lymphomas)
Tartrazine FD&C Yellow No.5 (E 102 Europe)	Allergies , Thyroid tumors, Lymphocytic lymphomas Trigger for asthma Urticaria (hives), Hyperactivity Chromosomal damage
Sunset Yellow FD&C Yellow No.6	Urticaria (hives), Rhinitis (runny nose) Nasal congestion, Allergies, Kidney tumors Bronchoconstriction (when combined with the Amaranth or Ponceau dyes), Anaphylactoid reaction (when combined with Ponceau), Distaste for food Eosinophilotactic response, Purpura, Chromosomal damage, Abdominal pain, Vomiting, Indigestion
Benomyl (a pesticide)	Decreased sperm count
BHA/BHT (petroleum-based preservatives found in meat, pastries and packaged foods)	Behavioral disturbances, Asthma attacks May cause cancer and liver ailments
Bromacil (a pesticide)	Thyroid/liver changes
Nitrates/Nitrites (preservatives found in many meat products; Canada banned their use in fish)	Potentially fatal toxic reactions in humans Carcinogenic effects
Fast Green, FD&C Green No.3	Bladder tumors
Brilliant Blue FD&C Blue No.1	Bronchoconstriction (when combined with the Erythrosine or Indigo Carmine dyes), Eosinophilotactic response, Chromosomal damage
Indigo Carmine FD&C Blue No.2	Brain tumors

*Information in this chart was compiled from:
1. The Feingold Association of the United States, "Adverse Effects of 'Inactive' Ingredients," www.feingold.org/effects.html.
2. Val Valerian, *The Psycho-Social, Chemical, Biological and Electromagnetic Manipula-*

Dropping Synthetics, Raising Test Scores
Children with ADHD aren't the only ones affected by food additives; I think the following experiment speaks volumes. In the fall of 1979, New York City schools made an innovative change in the district's lunch program: they excluded foods with high sugar content, as well as those containing two particular synthetic coloring agents. Within one year, the district's scores on standardized achievement tests showed an 8 percent increase in "mean academic percentile ranking." The school system then banned all synthetic food colorings and flavorings. The district's percentile ranking rose another 4 percent. In 1983, all foods containing the preservatives BHA and BHT were removed from school lunches. The school's rank increased an additional 4 percent.[9] Pretty impressive statistics if you ask me!

Eat Organic
Eating organic foods is the best way to ensure you avoid synthetic chemicals. Contrary to what some people believe, preservatives don't keep you "well-preserved." You may get away with eating the "Standard American Diet" (how S.A.D. it is!) while you're young, but check out older people; the majority have lost their zest along with their skin tone. Compare them to seniors who've been eating "health food" for decades and you'll really see the difference. Eating real, old-fashioned organic food is an investment that pays some serious dividends.

Aspartame

You might want to think twice before reaching for that diet six-pack. Check the label—see the word "aspartame?" You probably will, since it's an ingredient in almost all sugar-free products. As an artificial sweetener, aspartame is used in over 4,000 products worldwide, including some vitamin supplements. It is marketed as a diet aid, even though

tion of Human Consciousness (Volume I), Leading Edge Research Group, 1992. P.O. Box 2370, Yelm, WA 98597. www.trufax.org
3. Intnl. Food Information Council Foundation, www.ific.org.
4. Louise Tenney, *The Encyclopedia of Natural Remedies*, (Woodland Publishing, 2000), page 210.

research has shown that it causes the brain to stop producing serotonin, which results in feeling as though you haven't had enough to eat—even when full!

Virtually all scientific and anecdotal evidence available—except from those studies funded by groups which would benefit from the sale of aspartame—indicate that this additive is an extremely potent excitotoxin and is responsible for a myriad of health problems, especially in the nervous system.

Excitotoxins are substances that over-stimulate neurons and cause brain damage in varying degrees. Damage caused by these additives is not usually dramatic and in most instances the effects are subtle, cumulative, and develop over a prolonged period of time. However, more serious and instantaneous symptoms are also possible. Aspartame complaints to the FDA have included reports of headache, nausea, vertigo, insomnia, loss of limb control, blurred vision, blindness, memory loss, slurred speech, mild to severe depression, suicidal tendencies, hyperactivity, gastrointestinal disorders, seizures, skin lesions, rashes, anxiety attacks, muscle and joint pain, numbness, mood changes, menstrual cramps out of cycle, hearing loss or ringing in the ears, loss or change of taste, and symptoms similar to those of a heart attack.[1]

Russell L. Blaylock, M.D., author of: *Excitotoxins, The Taste That Kills*, states: "In my book on excitotoxins,[2] I explain in detail how these substances damage the nervous system, leading to severe disorders, and what can be done to reduce your risk. It is my opinion that aspartame is a dangerous neurotoxin, as well as a significant carcinogen for many organs, and should be avoided at all cost."[3]

Excitotoxins have also been shown to stimulate the generation of free radicals, which can have a negative impact on tissues and organs outside the central nervous system. Evidence indicates that free radical production accelerates many degenerative illnesses such as atherosclerosis, coronary artery disease and arthritis. Joint pain is a major complaint among those who have reported adverse reactions to aspartame.

In 1991, the National Institutes of Health listed 167 symptoms and reasons not to use aspartame. Studies of the additive in peer reviewed medical literature were surveyed for funding source and study outcome. Of the 166 studies felt to have relevance for questions of human safety, 74 had NutraSweet-related funding and 92 were independently funded.

One hundred percent (100%) of the industry-funded research attested to aspartame's safety, whereas 92 percent of the independently funded research identified problems.[4]

Scientifically known as 1-aspartyl 1-phenylalanine methyl ester, aspartame has three components: phenylalanine (50 percent), aspartic acid (40 percent) and methanol, also termed wood alcohol (10 percent). Phenylalanine and aspartic acid are amino acids that are normally supplied by the foods we eat; however, they can only be considered natural and harmless when consumed in combination with other amino acids. On their own, they enter the central nervous system in abnormally high concentrations, causing aberrant neuronal firing and probable cell death. The effects of these amino acids, when consumed as isolates, can be linked to headaches, mental confusion, balance problems and possibly seizures. Potentially more worrisome is that 10 percent of aspartame is absorbed into the bloodstream as methanol (wood alcohol). The Environmental Protection Agency defines safe consumption of methanol as no more than 7.8 milligrams per day. A one-liter beverage, sweetened with aspartame, contains about 56 milligrams of wood alcohol—*eight times* the EPA limit.

Aspartame's breakdown products, or metabolites, present an even greater cause for concern than its components. Phenylalanine decomposes into diketopiperazine (DKP), a known carcinogen when exposed to warm temperatures or prolonged storage. And even at cool or cold temperatures, methanol will spontaneously give rise to formaldehyde (a colorless toxin used as an embalming agent). Independent studies have shown formaldehyde formation resulting from aspartame ingestion to be extremely common. It accumulates within the cells, and reacts with cellular proteins such as enzymes and DNA. This cumulative reaction could spell grave consequences for those who consume aspartame-laden diet drinks and foods on a daily basis.[5]

Furthermore, infants are four times more sensitive to excitotoxins than are adults. During the first year of life, irreversible brain damage can occur through tainted agents in breast milk. *Despite this, the American Dietetic Association still recommends aspartame for pregnant and nursing women.*

The United States Air Force, though, recognizes its dangers. The May, 1992 issue of their official publication, *Flying Safety*, stated: "In pregnancy the effects of aspartame can be passed directly on to the fetus, even in very small doses." Both the U. S. Air Force and Navy have warned pilots about adverse reactions that can come from using aspartame products. Since some people have suffered aspartame-related disorders with doses as small as that contained in a single stick of chewing gum, this could mean that a pilot who drinks diet sodas is more susceptible to flicker vertigo, or to flicker-induced epileptic activity. Since 1988, over 600 pilots have complained about aspartame to the Aspartame Consumer Safety Network (www.aspartamesafety.com), an organization devoted to exposing the dangers of aspartame to the public.[6]

The FDA approved aspartame for use in food in 1974; that approval was revoked after it was shown to cause brain tumors in rats. In 1981, several FDA members who had opposed the use of aspartame vacated their positions. When those positions were filled, the new members re-approved aspartame for general consumption. There is convincing evidence that G.D. Searle, the original manufacturer and purveyor of aspartame, manipulated its testing of aspartame to get FDA approval,[7] and that the new management of the FDA was well aware of this.[8]

Check out these details (directly quoted from an article by Phil McDonald, reprinted at www.dorway.com/lethal.html): "On Jan 10, 1977, FDA Chief Counsel Richard Merrill recommended to U.S. attorney Sam Skinner, 'We request that your office convene a Grand Jury investigation into apparent violations of the Federal Food, Drug, and Cosmetic Act, and the False Reports to the Government Act, by G.D. Searle and Company and three of its responsible officers for their willful and knowing failure to make reports to the Food and Drug Administration, and for concealing material facts and making false statements in reports of animal studies conducted to establish the safety of the drug Aldactone and the food additive Aspartame.'"

Why was Searle not indicted? Searle's law firm, Sidney and Austin, met with attorney Skinner on January 26. A week later they offered him a job. On April 17, the Justice Department advised Skinner to proceed immediately because of a looming statute of limitations deadline. On July 1, Skinner switched sides to work for Sidney and Austin. His successor, attorney William Conlon, after convening a grand jury, let the statute of limitations run out on the aspartame charges. Fifteen months later he, too, went to work for Sidney and Austin. In all, TEN ranking

FDA or federal officials involved with the investigation and regulation of aspartame left government service for employment by the substitute sweetener industry."[9]

In 1980, the FDA created a Public Board of Inquiry to determine whether or not aspartame should be allowed onto the market. The board consisted of Peter J. Lampart, M.D., Professor and Chairman of the Department of Pathology at UCLA San Diego, Vernon R. Young, Ph.D., from the University of Nutritional Biochemistry at MIT, and Dr. Walle Nauta, Institute Professor at the Department of Psychology and Brain Science at MIT. They voted unanimously to recommend banning aspartame for human consumption.[10] But as surely as you see NutraSweet for sale today, the board's recommendation was never heeded.

In 1985, St. Louis-based Monsanto Corporation bought C.G. Searle. Monsanto manufactures pesticides, herbicides and other toxic chemicals. Monsanto also manufactures and markets Celebrex, which is promoted as a pain reliever for arthritis. Considering that their other products (pesticides and aspartame) may cause arthritis and significant health-related problems, and that they now market an arthritis drug, it appears they've cornered the market for pain and suffering—providing the cause and the band-aid to cover it.

DORway (www.dorway.com), one of many Web sites that exposes the dangers of aspartame, thinks it knows why: "Monsanto and the FDA would like you to believe that the entire media and medical system is pure as the driven snow... and that those of us exposing the dangers of aspartame are 'Toxic Terrorists' (CNN), or that we are weaving a 'WEB of Deceit' (TIME). Every last one of them has a vested interest in aspartame remaining a popular product. Monsanto has a billion dollars in sales annually, while the media has tens of billions of dollars invested in advertisements for over 5,000 products that contain aspartame. The medical system has hundreds of billions of dollars in expensive but useless tests that can't pinpoint patients' problems with certainty. Then, there are the many expensive drugs that don't seem to get the job done."

Even the National Soft Drink Association has expressed concern over the use of aspartame in soda pop. In 1983, they drafted a 30-page protest that was entered into the congressional record two years later. The draft included these words: "G. D. Searle and Company has not demonstrated to a certainty that the use of aspartame in soft drinks... will not adversely affect human health as a result of the changes such use is likely to cause in brain chemistry."[11]

So, now you know. For vibrant health, avoid aspartame and other synthetic sweeteners. An alternative to aspartame (or sugar for that matter) is the herb stevia, which is completely safe. Unfortunately, the FDA has made it *illegal* for manufacturers of stevia to state that it's a sugar substitute (they even tried to burn books about stevia—but that's another story)! After all, if the public knew of a sugar substitute that was not only calorie free, but completely safe, our choice would be easy. But that would not be in their best interests.

Sugar

"I am confident that Western medicine will admit what has been known in the Orient for years: sugar is without question the number one murderer in the history of humanity—much more lethal than opium or radioactive fallout."[1]

Nyoiti Sakurazawa, Japanese Doctor

"No matter how difficult it is to realize that something so sweet can really be the devil in disguise, we have to start believing it. The hard facts are staring us in the face and telling us in no uncertain terms that our health and lives depend upon it."[2]

Ann Louise Gittleman, M.S., C.N.S.

The statements above may seem radical, but refined sugar, so seductive and sweet, is also an addictive poison. Heavily processed, it lacks nutritional value and saps minerals from the body. It is linked to health problems that go well beyond obesity. My advice: avoid it. We'll discuss some healthy alternatives after examining some of the facts about refined sugar.

The Addiction Risk

Many holistic healers insist that refined sugar is addictive, a view examined by the mainstream scientific community at a summer 2003 conference, when Princeton University researchers induced lab rats to binge on large amounts of sugar and then abruptly excluded it from the animals' diets. The rats experienced withdrawal-like symptoms: their teeth chattered, they became anxious and the usual balance of neurochemicals in the parts of their brains pertaining to motive was turned upside-down.[3]

Sweet Poison?

Natural health advocates who allege that sugar is a poison are largely following in the footsteps of William Coda Martin, a doctor who expressed early support for this view. In a 1957 article published in the *Michigan Organic News*, he wrote that: "Medically, poison denotes any substance applied to, ingested or developed within the body that causes or may cause disease." Physically, he defined poison as "any substance that inhibits the activity of chemical or enzymatic catalysts that activate a reaction." He included refined sugar, which is transformed into pure, refined carbohydrates, as being such a substance. He explained that the body cannot utilize this refined starch and carbohydrate unless proteins, vitamins and minerals are present.

Nature supplies these elements in each plant in quantities sufficient to metabolize the carbohydrate in that particular plant. There is no excess for added carbohydrates. Incomplete carbohydrate metabolism results in the formation of 'toxic metabolites' such as pyruvic acid and abnormal sugars containing five carbon atoms. Pyruvic acid accumulates in the brain and nervous system, while abnormal sugars accumulate in red blood cells. These toxic metabolites interfere with the respiration of the cells, which cannot get sufficient oxygen to survive and function normally. In time, some of the cells die. This, he concludes, "interferes with the function of a part of the body and is the beginning of degenerative disease."[4]

B Vitamin Depletion

When you eat refined sugar, you ingest a substance that not only lacks nutritional value, but also robs your body of minerals (such as chromium, manganese, cobalt, copper, zinc and magnesium), enzymes and vitamins (especially the B vitamins). B vitamins are required to metabolize sugar. Constant sugar consumption can lead to a vitamin B deficiency, which translates into poor metabolism, low energy and mental/nervous disorders. Many B vitamins (which are responsible for proper nerve and brain function) are manufactured by symbiotic bacteria living in our intestines. Too much refined sugar kills these friendly bacteria, resulting in an even greater B vitamin deficiency, which can cause sleepiness, mental fatigue and many other symptoms. Furthermore, a significant loss of friendly bacteria in the gut allows entry of unfriendly bacteria, which can weaken the immune system (and often leads to ear infections, particularly in children).

Daily intake of refined sugar creates an acidic condition that quickly consumes the body's minerals—especially calcium, needed to alkalinize the system—causing a general weakening of the body. The parasympathetic nervous system, which governs our digestive processes, is adversely affected; thus, food cannot be digested or assimilated properly. This leads to a blood sugar imbalance and an intensified craving for sugar—hence, one component of addiction.

Refined sugar passes quickly into the bloodstream in large amounts, which shocks the pancreas and stomach. The pancreas goes into overdrive to make enough insulin (a hormone that carries sugar to the cells to be metabolized or stored) to normalize blood sugar by taking excess sugar out of the bloodstream and turning it into glycogen for energy or moving it into fat storage. This can cause a sudden drop in blood sugar, which then signals the adrenal glands to release high levels of cortisol (the fight or flight hormone), putting the body into high-stress mode. The result is a quick burst of energy that lasts about two hours, followed by an equally fast drop in energy. Picks you up and lets you down!

The Hypoglycemia & Diabetes Connection

Hypoglycemia and adult-onset diabetes are directly linked to sugar consumption—there are estimates that 98 percent of all adult-onset diabetes is diet-induced. Hypoglycemia occurs when refined sugar and/or other refined foods such as white flour, are consumed on a regular basis. Hypoglycemia is a state of low blood sugar due to an over-reactive pancreas that sends out too much insulin to compensate for the excess processed sugar. Symptoms of hypoglycemia include fatigue, lack of concentration, anxiety, mood swings and irritability. Adult-onset diabetes usually follows hypoglycemia when insulin receptors in the cells no longer respond to the insulin being produced by the pancreas, causing high blood sugar and/or when insulin production has dropped or stopped. These degenerative diseases are virtually always diet-related and are completely avoidable (and reversible)!

Immune System Suppression

Refined sugar also slowly destroys the immune system by:

- Undermining the ability of white blood cells to kill germs for up to five hours after ingestion
- Reducing the production of antibodies
- Interfering with the transport of vitamin C (an important immune builder)
- Causing severe mineral imbalances
- Neutralizing the action of essential fatty acids

Since our immune system is involved in every aspect of maintaining health, the over-consumption of sugar may be linked to virtually every known ailment and degenerative disease.

Joseph Mercola, DO, with Nancy Applegate, author of *Lick the Sugar Habit*, has compiled an extraordinary list of 78 reasons to avoid sugar, gleaned from an array of scientific and medical literature. The list, with its carefully cited claims, is damning; it indicts sugar for a host of modern ailments, including varicose veins, depression, increased risk of Alzheimer's disease, asthma, arthritis, cataracts, etc. And, of course, the two health risks you already knew went hand in hand with sugar—tooth decay and obesity. For the complete list with citations, see: www.mercola.com/article/sugar/dangers_of_sugar.htm

Avoiding refined sugar can be tricky, because it's in nearly everything we eat and drink. The average American consumes 150 pounds of refined sweeteners each year. For example, most soda pop has at least seven teaspoons worth of refined sugar per can. You have to know how to translate the ingredients on labels, because refined sugar has many names, depending on its source. When derived from sugar cane or beets, it's called sucrose; when derived from corn it's called dextrose. It's known as fructose when derived from fruit and as maltose when derived from malt.

Artificial Sweeteners

I'd like to stress that substituting artificial sweeteners for refined sugar is not the way to go. Many such sweeteners have been associated with serious health problems—so why take the risk, especially when, as you'll see below, you have plenty of other options? When assessing the hazards of artificial sweeteners, consider aspartame, commonly sold under the trade names NutraSweet and Equal, approved by the FDA in the early 1980s amid controversy. Since its approval, some health organizations— even those that vouch for its safety—have acknowledged an extraordinary number of public complaints, recorded but largely dismissed by the FDA, about aspartame's neurotoxic side-effects. Check out the thorough discussion of aspartame earlier in this chapter for more details.

Healthy Alternatives

There are several alternative sweeteners that are much healthier than refined sugar. Pure maple syrup contains minerals and vitamins, as do blackstrap molasses, rice syrup and barley malt. All of these sweeteners can be found at natural foods stores. When you have a sweet tooth and want to buy a prepackaged product, look for those that contain one of these natural sweeteners instead of refined sugars or anything ending in "ose." At a natural foods store, you can even find soda pop with less sugar (or with "better" sweeteners, as listed above) than their conventional counterparts.

Stevia

Another alternative sweetener that contains no calories and improves digestion is the herb stevia, which is about 200 times sweeter than sugar. Unfortunately, the FDA has outlawed manufacturers of stevia from labeling it as an alternative sweetener, so stevia is marketed as a supplement. Although stevia is a completely safe herb that has been used for thousands of years, the FDA, citing a lack of conclusive studies on the herb's safety, banned its sale in the United States in the early 1990s, until the natural foods industry got it approved as a supplement.

Companies are eager to use stevia as a natural sweetener, but can't afford the price and hassle of ignoring the FDA's stance. By 2001, stevia sales reached $10 million in the United States; however, no company marketing the herb is equal to the financial might of G.D. Searle, the pharmaceutical firm that pushed for FDA approval of aspartame. (Interestingly, Searle was later bought out by Monsanto, which in 2000 sold its sweetener business for $440 million cash[5]).

In the late 1990s, Stevita, a Texas-based company that has produced and sold stevia for 15 years, was targeted by the FDA for allegedly marketing its products as sweeteners. FDA agents entered the company's warehouses, looking for "labeling violations," books and other material representing stevia as a conventional food product. After sifting through various printed materials, the agency determined the company had violated the Federal Food, Drug, and Cosmetic Act of 1997. Stevita's President and Vice-Presidents have said that the FDA ordered the destruction of stevia-related publications, a claim the FDA denies. But the agency does not deny expending substantial time and effort (and consequently, money) to carry out detailed inspections of Stevita's and other companies' warehouses, as well as of retail establishments—a shining example of your tax dollars at work.

Stevia is a threat to both the sugar and artificial sweetening industries, so it's no wonder the FDA has done all it can to stop the sale of this remarkable herbal sweetener. But don't let them stop you from trying it. You can get it in packets just like Equal and NutraSweet, or in liquid form. The small bottle seems expensive, but you only need a drop or two. Check out www.cookingwithstevia.com for more stevia facts and recipes, as well as a stevia-to-sugar conversion chart (unlike aspartame, which loses its sweetness at high temperatures, stevia can be used in cooking).

Refined Oils and Salt

"One hundred years ago, heart disease was virtually unknown. Today, two-thirds of US citizens develop heart disease. Something has clearly gone wrong with the way we are living, and one of the main factors may well be the introduction of refined, over-processed, devitalized oils."[1]
–Dr. Dane Roubos, B.Sc., D.C.

When you shop at the supermarket and buy conventional, non-organic produce or pre-packaged foods, you risk being exposed to a multitude of poisons in minute quantities. Most conventional packaged foods have been so processed that all the natural vitamins, minerals and life force have been stripped away, leaving you with virtual "non-foods," which then require artificial flavorings and colorings to be palatable. Instead of eating these food substitutes, (known in the industry as "designer foods") I suggest you buy only natural foods, preferably organic. Addi-

tionally, there are a few specific processed foods that ought to be entirely
eliminated from your diet, because they cause harm to the body.

Highly Processed Oils
Nearly all oils carried by conventional supermarkets have been processed
to such a degree that your health will be compromised if you ingest them
on a regular basis. The refining process usually includes using a chemical
solvent (often hexane) for extraction of the oil, and very high temperatures (of over 400 degrees) for processing and deodorizing. The resulting
oil—often colorless and nearly tasteless—is packed with newly formed
trans fatty acids, which are known to raise cholesterol levels in the blood
and cause metabolic disorders such as cancer and arthritis. Oils easily go
rancid, especially when stored in clear bottles; rancidity also contributes
to health problems. When these oils are used for cooking, even more
trans fatty acids are created, making a potentially hazardous meal!

The alternative is to buy "expeller pressed," unrefined, organic oils.
Expeller-pressed means the oil has been extracted mechanically rather
than via heat. Look for the word "unrefined" on the label, indicating that
the oil has not been subjected to high heat and thus retains its full flavor.
Even expeller-pressed, organic oils are subject to rancidity, so buy those
which come in dark bottles whenever possible (the darker bottle shields
the oil from light oxidation more than a clear bottle does).

In my opinion, the best oils for recipes and salads are olive and sesame. For cooking, unrefined coconut oil (hard at room temperature) is
the best. You read that right! Coconut oil has gotten a bad rap, mostly
because the soybean industry managed to convince the public through
a massive advertising campaign that heat or chemical processed coconut
oil contributes to high cholesterol. However, expeller pressed coconut oil
is a fantastic oil that can tolerate high cooking temperatures and it offers
numerous health benefits. It can kill viruses that cause influenza, hepati-
tis C, measles, herpes and even AIDS, as well as bacteria, fungi and yeast,
while boosting energy and improving digestion.[2] Flaxseed oil, because of
its high omega 3 and omega 6 fatty acid content, is also excellent for salads and baked goods, but never use this oil for cooking (see the Supplement chapter for more information about flax oil, and the Appendix for
how I use it on most of my food).

Margarine

Many people buy margarine to avoid using butter. Unfortunately, margarine is created by a process called hydrogenation. This process adds hydrogen to an oil to make it hard at room temperature, but creates an immune-damaging synthetic fat—a type of trans fatty acid. As stated before, trans fatty acids elevate blood cholesterol, which can cause health problems such as heart disease. Trans-fatty acids in cell membranes weaken the membrane's protective structure and function. This alters normal transport of minerals and other nutrients across the membrane and allows disease microbes and toxic chemicals to get into the cell more easily. The result: sick, weakened cells, poor organ function and an exhausted immune system. In the United States, 95 percent of trans fatty ingestion is from eating margarine and shortening.[3] Be aware of hydrogenated (or partially hydrogenated) oils in packaged foods and avoid them completely. *Margarine is basically a non-food.*

Fortunately, an all-natural margarine-like product called Earth Balance Natural Buttery Spread is now available. It's GMO-free, 100 percent expeller pressed, is not hydrogenated and contains no animal products. I eat it all the time and believe it's currently the best product on the market.

Salt

The effect of salt on body chemistry is not well understood by many people. Most of us believe that salt is bad for our health and that we need to reduce our intake of it. However, this isn't exactly true. While *refined* salt *is* bad for us, sea salt in its natural form is actually beneficial. And since potassium is the regulator of sodium chloride (salt), it's when our *potassium/sodium ratio* is out of balance that salt is detrimental.

Sea salt (in its natural, unrefined form) has been considered essential for good health for aeons. In the sixth century, merchants traded it with the equivalent value of gold. Salt was used as payment to Roman soldiers, which is where we get the word *salary*. For centuries the French were required to buy their salt from royal despots; the tax was so high that it helped ignite the French Revolution. In 1930, in protest against the high tax imposed on salt in India by the British Government, Mahatma Gandhi led a mass pilgrimage of his followers to the seaside to make their own salt (which was an illegal act according to British law).[4] If salt was so important to our health back then, why is it so unpopular today? Over-processing has changed a natural, necessary element into a chemical, synthetic imitation.

Over 65 years ago, salt manufacturers sped up production by drying salt in huge kilns which could reach temperatures of 1,200 degrees. This process not only changes the chemical structure of salt, but also completely eliminates about 4 percent of its mixed trace mineral content. In fact, over 60 trace minerals are virtually wiped out by the processing. What's left is a chemical structure of about 99.5 percent sodium chloride, to which anti-caking chemicals, potassium iodide and dextrose (sugar) are added to stabilize the iodine. The result is a new chemical structure, which corporations label as salt, but in reality is an entirely different component—one that doesn't agree with the body.[5]

As I already mentioned, the amount of salt retained in our bodies is primarily controlled by the metabolic action of potassium in relationship to sodium, known as the *sodium/potassium ratio*. When the ratio is balanced, the body retains the amount of salt it requires and discards the rest. When this balance is not maintained, then salt (sodium chloride) can cause health problems.

Potassium is a nutrient essential to our health, but is rarely found in processed foods. Furthermore, foods such as coffee, alcohol, candy and sweets deplete potassium supplies in our body. Eating refined foods that are high in sodium with little to no potassium strongly contributes to high blood pressure, cardiovascular problems and degenerative diseases. To summarize, eating sodium chloride in place of natural, unprocessed salt and depleting our potassium levels causes the health problems that are blamed on too much salt!

Unrefined sea salt, on the other hand, is quite beneficial in reasonable quantities. It's still a good idea to read the labels for salt content, even on natural food products. Unrefined sea salt (which has a gray hue) contains approximately 4 percent trace minerals—a profile similar to that of our blood (hence its popularity and value for thousands of years). Sea salt has a purifying effect on toxic residues in foods; it strengthens digestion and contributes to the secretion of hydrochloric acid in the stomach. Sea salt also helps build the immune system. Most diseases gain foothold in an acidic body, and sea salt helps to neutralize that condition by making us more alkaline. As I said, about 60 trace minerals are found in sea salt.

Interestingly, vitamins cannot work properly without minerals.

Sea salt also contributes to solid mental health and emotional stability. Whereas refined sugar (and sweets in general) has an overly expansive effect on consciousness (known as "yin" in Macrobiotics), sea salt—because of its mineral content—has a very grounding effect (known as "yang" in Macrobiotics). [See Chapter 5 for a more detailed discussion of the yin/yang concept and of acid/alkaline conditions in the body.]

Avoid refined salt entirely, both at home and in packaged goods—it's just not good for you. Using sea salt and eating unrefined, whole, organic foods—which contain large quantities of potassium—*is* good for you. You can buy unrefined sea salt at natural foods stores. Look for larger crystals that are a little gray in color. If they aren't gray, the salt may have been processed to some degree. Another excellent source of sea salt is seaweed. My favorite seaweed to add to soups and other cooked meals is dulse. It has a mild flavor and is a great source for sea salt and minerals.

Monosodium Glutamate (MSG)

"MSG is a drug added to our foods that
causes widespread toxicity."[1]
–George R. Schwartz, M.D.
In Bad Taste–The MSG Symptom Complex

In many Philippine provinces, as in the rest of Asia, it is not uncommon for people to eat dogs, after poisoning them with one or two tablespoons of monosodium glutamate (MSG) placed inside a roll of bread. The dog salivates, loses consciousness and involuntarily spasms until breathing stops.[2]

MSG is a drug. It has no flavor of its own and synthetically enhances the taste of food by altering the way the tongue, nervous system and brain communicate with one another. It intensifies the flavor of savory foods by causing neuron cells in the mouth to over-react to different flavors. Unfortunately, these over-stimulated cells exhaust themselves and die, causing microscopic scarring throughout the human system.[3] Within 30 minutes of eating processed foods high in MSG, neurons swell up like balloons and die after three hours. With lower doses, neuron cells die after 18 to 24 hours.[4]

Yet, you'll find MSG in the spice section of your local supermarket. It's in many seasoning mixes and is used in most processed foods—candy, cakes, donuts, dairy products, snack foods, frozen entrées, salad dressings and soups, to name a few. It is often disguised under different names, such as hydrolyzed protein, sodium caseinate or calcium caseinate, gelatin, textured protein, carrageenan or vegetable gum. Still more is hidden in flavorings of all kinds (including chicken, beef, pork, smoke and even "natural" flavorings), bouillon, broth or stock, malt extract, malt

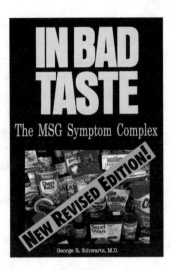

flavoring, whey protein, whey protein isolate or concentrate, soy protein, soy protein isolate or concentrate, soy sauce or extract, "zest," "gourmet powder," and more.[5]

MSG was first developed in Japan in 1909, and soon gained widespread acceptance in the Orient. In 1948, it was introduced to the American food industry as a flavor enhancer for otherwise bland food products, during a national convention in Chicago, attended by all the major food producers, including Campbell Foods, Continental Foods, General Foods, Nestles, United Airline Food Service, Libbey, Pillsbury and Oscar Mayer.[6]

In a 1974 questionnaire, Dr. Liane Reif-Lehrer, a noted researcher at Harvard Medical School, investigated people's reactions to MSG. Almost 30 percent of the 1,529 respondents reported dizziness, nausea, abdominal pain, visual disturbances, fatigue, shortness of breath, weakness, headache or tightness around the face. Emotional reactions ranged from depression and insomnia to "feeling tense."[7]

More than 500 million people worldwide and approximately 5 percent of Americans react severely to very small amounts of MSG, and up to 30 percent have a noticeable reaction. Many scientists and researchers label MSG as a neurotoxin and suggest that it may contribute to Alzheimer's and Lou Gehrig's Disease, Huntington's Chorea, Parkinson's Disease and other neurological diseases.

A reaction may be caused by as little as 1/10th of a teaspoonful (1/2 gram). Many packaged meals contain three grams or more. Common reactions include dizziness, headache, flushing and burning sensations.[8] The more we ingest, the greater the reaction, which in rare instances is fatal. Infants, senior citizens, asthmatics, people with neurological and immune disease health challenges, heart or digestive tract problems and severe mood or depression problems are most at risk.

More than 10 years ago psychiatrist Dr. John Olney from Washington University in St. Louis said during a neuroscience meeting that, "Over 20 years ago [over 30 now] glutamate was shown to cause brain damage to infant animals. Since then, it has become increasingly evident that glutamate and closely related substances are neurotoxins that can cause human neuro-degenerative diseases."[9] Dr. Olney conducted studies on rodents and found that MSG damaged the hypothalamus gland. It also caused obesity, behavioral and endocrine changes, stunted bodies and caused seizures and infertility. Hypothalamic neurons responsible for growth regulation, puberty onset, memory and learning, endocrine functions, appetite and circadian rhythms were destroyed.[10] He also discovered that children typically get enough MSG in one bowl of commercial soup to raise blood glutamate levels to those found to cause severe brain cell damage in experimental animals.[11]

MSG is never safe—even if you don't react to it. Avoiding all forms of MSG is the best choice for those who desire vibrant health.

3
Food
Embrace Organic

Most of the food we eat is compromised in one way or another, creating a plethora of degenerative diseases and health problems. Twelve years of research on the subject has convinced me that a consistent diet of chemically "enhanced," highly processed and nutritionally deficient food is the number one cause of chronic health problems in this country. Of course, there can be reasons other than diet to account for poor health. However, good nutrition *is* one of the keys to good health, and I believe it is the continuous ingestion of micro amounts of toxins, combined with *inadequate nutrition,* that has created such an epidemic of obesity and degenerative disease among Americans.

It's no mystery that nutrition is a critical link to health; yet mainstream culture (and even mainstream medicine) chooses to minimize or ignore that fact. As a result, fast-food and junk food purveyors are reaping high profits. Most doctors treat disease without even discussing nutrition with their patients. Therefore, I want to help you eat in a way that encourages good health. You must break with mainstream thinking and develop alternative habits, and the best and most effective way to avoid problem-causing devitalized and chemically "enhanced" food is to eat organically grown food.

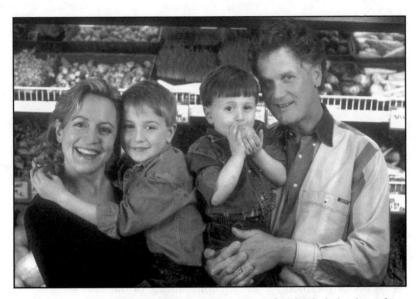

"Chemically produced foods are dangerous for the little bodies of children. Nature intends for us to eat pure food—so we eat organically grown foods. We all feel 100% better now that we eat organic."

—Donna Stewart

Why Organic?

You'll want to stock only organically grown food in your home because it is the least toxic, best tasting, most nutrient-dense food available. Organically grown food is not genetically modified or irradiated and is free of synthetic pesticides, herbicides, preservatives and additives. When used in packaged products, organic food is usually minimally processed to maintain its integrity. Organic food is grown using farming techniques that maintain and replenish the fertility of the soil by working in harmony with nature instead of against it. Organic food is grown without the use of toxic and persistent pesticides or herbicides, and without sewage sludge fertilizers, which often contain highly toxic "recycled" heavy metals and other pollutants.

Organic farmers understand that soil is the very body of the Earth, and therefore they create an ecosystem of living organisms in the soil. On the other hand, farmers who use synthetic chemicals to control weeds and pests create soil devoid of the worms and microorganisms needed to keep it naturally aerated and fertile. It's a dead ecosystem because these chemicals and management techniques work to control and conquer life, rather than replenish it. Dead soil means minimal nutrition for plants and, therefore, minimal nutrition for us. As we learned earlier, conventionally grown plants can absorb toxic pesticides and herbicides, which can be passed on to us when we eat them.

Organic farms, on the other hand, use live soil—teeming with worms and microorganisms—which help plants absorb nutrients and therefore *naturally* ward off insects and disease. When pesticides or herbicides are required, organic farmers use compounds that are minimally toxic to humans and non-persistent (they dissipate quickly).

When you purchase organic foods, you're supporting a complete environment and people-friendly agricultural system that:

- Reduces the amount of toxic chemicals in our food supply,
- Protects the health of future generations by creating long-term solutions to agricultural problems,
- Uses practices that eliminate polluting chemicals, thus protecting and conserving our water resources,
- Supports farmers who replenish and maintain soil fertility, and
- Builds biologically diverse agriculture.

Eating only organically grown foods at home guarantees that you are eating pure food as often as possible. Since most restaurants don't use organic food, what you stock at home is all important. Organic food is more costly than conventionally grown food because it is more labor intensive to produce. But paying extra money now for top-of-the-line food could easily translate into money saved from potential medical bills later. For more specific information on the nutritional and environmental benefits of eating organically grown food, visit the Organic Consumer's Association Web site at www.organicconsumers.org.

Where to Find It
Organic food can be purchased from a variety of sources. Prices for organic food can be high or low, depending on where you buy it. Some outlets are more expensive than others, and if you have a family to feed, you may want to check into the lower priced options first.

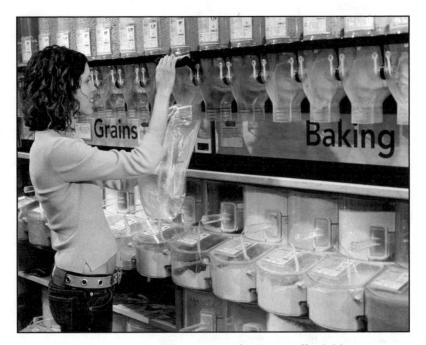

Buying in bulk makes organic food very affordable.

Community Supported Agriculture (CSA)

Community Supported Agriculture (CSA) is a system which allows you to have a direct relationship with a farmer during the growing season. Generally, you pay the farmer at the beginning of the growing season (or sometimes throughout the growing season) and in return the farmer supplies you with food every week or every other week. Most farms participating in this program supply only organically grown food.

This arrangement provides benefits to both you and the farmer. You get a variety of organic food at a reduced price and the farmer has a steady income for producing food throughout the growing season. CSAs make eating organic food an affordable arrangement for large families on a budget. In fact, some farms even let their members help on the farm, which reduces the cost of organic food even more. It's a win/win situation for all involved.

To find a CSA near you, visit www.nal.usda.gov/afsic/csa/csastate. htm or talk with management at your local natural food store.

Farmers Markets

With over 3,100 farmers markets in the United States, it should be fairly easy to find one close by if you live in a major city. Similar to a CSA, you get to deal directly with the farmer or the farmer's representative, which benefits the farmer and you. The farmer makes a little more money selling directly to the end customer, and you often pay less for the food than you would at a retail store.

Not all farmers markets include produce from organic farms, but many do. If you like to get out and meet people, shopping for organic food at a farmers market is a great way to save money, get farm fresh produce and enjoy the sense of community and aliveness of an open market. Find one near you by visiting www.ams.usda.gov/farmersmarkets or talking with management at your local natural food store.

Organic Food Delivery

Most large cities now sport businesses that deliver organic food directly to your home or office once or twice a week. Sometimes you get to choose the type of produce to be delivered, but usually the assortment of produce is determined by the delivery service and the farms with which they are associated. Home delivery of organic produce is obviously more expensive than leaving home to get it, but if you lead a busy lifestyle, home delivery may be the answer for you. It's a convenient way to buy organic that more and more people are embracing. In fact, it has become so popular that many cities have more than one organic food delivery service. To find one near you, do a Google search on the Web ("organic delivery" and "your city"), look for advertisements in local alternative publications and talk with management at your local natural food store.

Natural Food Stores

Although some conventional grocery stores are finally carrying organic produce in limited quantities, natural food stores ("health food stores") devote most of their produce section to organic food. *You'll pay top dollar for organic produce at a conventional grocery store, and that is why many people believe it is so expensive.* However, although organic food certainly costs more than conventionally grown food, you'll find that overall it's less expensive when you shop at your local natural food store. Most large natural food stores carry a wide variety of organic produce all year long.

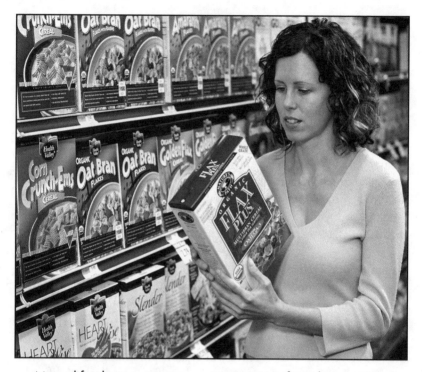

Natural food stores carry an organic version of nearly every type
of product you'd find at a conventional grocery store.

Natural food stores not only carry a large assortment of fresh organic
produce, but also carry a wide variety of boxed, canned or frozen foods
that are either all organic, or are at least devoid of synthetic chemicals and
additives. In fact, natural food stores carry not only healthy food options,
but also a wide variety of products devoted to the healthy lifestyle, such
as botanical health and beauty products, products made from recycled
resources, whole food supplements, natural healing remedies, non-toxic
biodegradable household cleaning products, and more. Shopping at a
natural food store is a rewarding experience that offers you access to some
of the highest quality health-enhancing products available today.

4
Grocery Shopping
Go to a Natural Food Store

If you're serious about buying organic food and living a healthier life-style, you'll eventually want to switch from shopping at a conventional grocery store to shopping at a natural food store (also known as a "health food store"). The reason is simple: natural food stores consciously stock products that are better for you and for the environment, and refuse to carry most products considered by natural living standards to be unhealthy. With over 8,000 such stores nationwide today, there is sure to be one near you—just look in the Yellow Pages under "Health Food Stores," consult *GreenPeople's* on-line database (www.greenpeople.org/healthfood. htm), or purchase the book *Healthy Highways* by David and Nikki Goldbeck to find over 1,900 natural food stores and health conscious restaurants.

Although some conventional grocery stores are finally carrying organic produce and natural products in limited quantities, you'll pay a higher price for them there than at the natural food store. Furthermore, the owners and management of conventional stores are often driven mainly by profits, while owners of natural food stores are driven by both profits and a philosophy. The philosophy is that we should only use products that are healthy for us and for the environment. Every business must make a profit to stay in business, but not necessarily at the expense of our health or the environment! The success of large natural food store chains such as Whole Foods and Wild Oats have proven that a business can

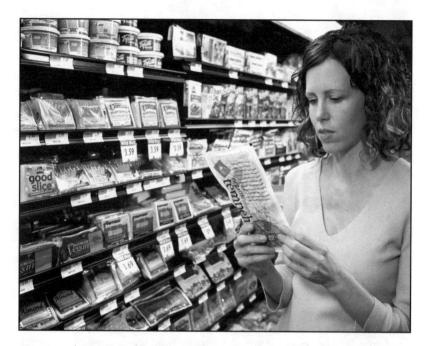

A wide variety of healthy, delicious food products are available
in natural food stores, but not conventional stores.

achieve success while remaining true to this philosophy.

Natural food stores carry not only a wide selection of organic produce, but also carry almost all the other types of products you would find
at a conventional store—only these products are more healthy for us and
the environment. Let's take a look at what's offered.

Natural Food

Not all the food carried in a natural food store is organic, but virtually all
of it, whether canned, frozen or boxed, is devoid of synthetic chemical
additives such as preservatives, synthetic food dyes, artificial flavorings
and the like. Often the products are minimally processed, so they don't
require the addition of synthetic vitamins, either. Usually these products
have a shorter shelf life, which is one reason why they cost a little more.
Personally, I think they are more nutritious and taste much better than
their conventional brand counterparts.

Most of the natural food products are carefully chosen by store management to ensure that the store stocks only nutritious—or at least nontoxic—food products. And there is a huge variety of natural food products to choose from, replacing virtually every type of product you would find in a conventional store. By buying natural and organic food at a natural food store, you minimize the amount of toxins you ingest. Better health is the long-term result.

You'll find a bulk food section at natural food stores, often with a substantial organic selection. If you have a large family, buying bulk items such as organic grains, beans and nuts is a great way to save money, yet eat healthy. You'll find multiple types of meat substitutes, as well as organic meat at most natural food stores. Conventional meat is often loaded with toxic chemicals such as pesticides, artificial growth hormones, artificial food additives, tranquilizers, antibiotics or disease-causing organisms.

Health & Beauty Products
Another great advantage of shopping at a natural food store is the wide variety of botanically based health and beauty products such as toothpaste, shampoo, make-up, skin creams, deodorant, bar soap, moisturizers and so on. What's different is that "natural" manufacturers use "botanical" (plant-based) ingredients in their products, instead of only synthetic chemical ingredients found in conventional beauty products.

What we put on our skin is absorbed into the body, for better or worse. Many researchers believe that consistent application of synthetic chemicals onto our skin can cause health problems. For example, aluminum is found in many conventional deodorant products, yet aluminum has been linked to breast cancer and Alzheimer's disease. Thus, you can find aluminum-free beauty products at natural food stores.

There is debate within the natural health and beauty product community as to whether or not *any* synthetic chemicals should be used in products labeled as "natural." Virtually all agree however, that the more botanics (e.g., plant derived) a product contains, the better it is for us. The reason is twofold: the product is less toxic (or nontoxic) than its synthetic counterpart, and the healing properties of the botanicals help rejuvenate, repair and/or improve our skin, hair, gums and teeth.

For example, many manufacturers—both conventional and natural—use fragrance oils in their products. Fragrance oils are synthetic

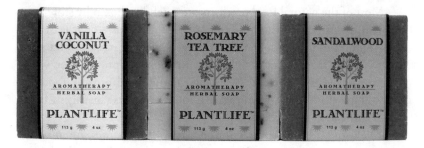

PlantLife Natural Body Care uses pure botanical ingredients.

(man made) and contain potentially harmful chemicals such as methylene chloride, toluene, methyl ethyl ketone, ethonal and others, yet have no redeeming value beyond the fragrance. On the other hand, pure essential oils—oils that are extracted from plants using special methods to retain their inherent qualities—not only offer delightful fragrances, but can provide ample medicinal value as well. One well-known essential oil, lavender oil, contains these therapeutic properties: antiseptic, antidepressant, anti-spasmodic, diuretic, sedative, insecticide; and it has a soothing effect on nerves. The bottom line? Pure botanical products often cost more because they're more expensive to produce, but, the more "botanical" the product is, the more therapeutic it's likely to be! And that's one of the main reasons to use these type of personal care products.

Another aspect of the personal care products found in health food stores is that most of these products have been manufactured in a way designed to retain as much of the medicinal value of the plant as possible. For example, all soap is made from plant oils, animal oils and/or synthetic chemicals, with plant oils being the most desirable. Most soap on the market is "milled." This means that the natural glycerin and good properties of the plant oils are removed from the soap, making it a harder bar soap that will last longer, but also dry out your skin. However, for soap that is cold-processed (a natural process), all the good properties of the plant oils and the natural occurring glycerin from the soap making process are retained. This means that cold-processed soap will leave the plant oils on your skin, providing you with the medicinal value of those oils.

I've been using all natural, 100% pure essential oil soap for quite some time now, and I can tell you first hand that that's the way to go! I'm happy to share with you that I have found and been using some of the very best all natural 100% pure essential oil soap available, manufactured by PlantLife Natural Body Care (www.PlantLife.net) In addition to the fact that their soaps are cold-processed and use 100% pure essential oils, PlantLife offers a (seemingly) endless number of essential oil variations of their soap to satisfy anyone's senses. I highly recommend their products and hope you'll give them a try. (To learn more about the medicinal value of pure essential oils, please visit page 163.)

Supplements & Healing Remedies

Natural food stores carry a very wide variety of supplements (for regular use), and natural healing remedies (for ailments). Whereas in conventional grocery stores you'll find a vast array of chemically produced "medicines" designed to manage symptoms, in natural food stores you'll find natural supplements and remedies formulated to work harmoniously with your body to help it rejuvenate and heal. Because there are an almost overwhelming number of products to choose from, Chapters 6 and 10 provide an overview of the essential supplements and remedies I recommend.

Products Made From Recycled Resources

Most paper products available from conventional stores—paper plates, napkins, bathroom tissue, paper towels, sanitary pads and even diapers—are not only made from virgin resources, but have been bleached with chlorine, a source of dangerous toxins such as dioxin, furans and other organochlorines. On the other hand, natural food stores stock natural paper products created from recycled resources that have been whitened without the use of highly toxic chlorine bleach. Yes, they cost slightly more, but they are better for you and help preserve the environment. Of particular note are diapers and feminine products that are in constant contact with the skin. Especially in these cases, using non-toxic, dioxin-free products from recycled resources is your best bet for comfort, reliability and health.

Deli "Fast Food" & Café

Many natural food stores sport a refrigerated section stocked with a variety of pre-made sandwiches, wraps, rice dishes and other wholesome

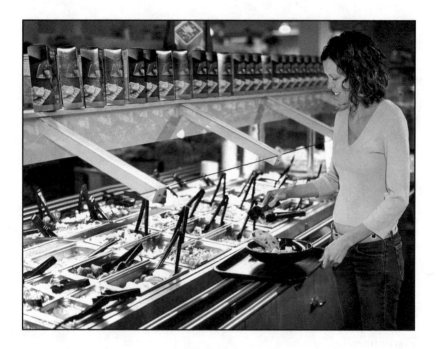

foods. Some even offer a full-blown deli and/or salad bar with a wide selection of hot menu items. When you're in a hurry, forget the fast food
joint and instead go to your local natural food store to find a nutritious,
and delicious, meal.

Non-Toxic Cleaning Products

Cleaning products include dish soaps, laundry detergents, bathroom cleaners and similar household cleaning products. Most conventional cleaning
products rely on harsh, and usually toxic, petroleum-based chemicals to
do their job. These conventional cleaning products are poisonous to humans and the environment, and they can cause serious damage to our
health. On the other hand, natural cleaning products rely primarily on
plant-based ingredients to do their job, which makes them virtually non-
toxic to humans and the environment. Over a half million children under
the age of 6 are poisoned every year in their homes. Sheer safety consider-
ations are reason enough to use non-toxic cleaning supplies.

Maybe you're now asking the question, "Do they work?" My answer

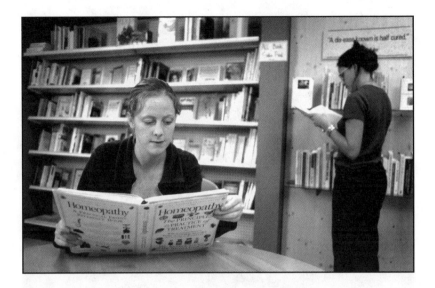

Some of the best books on natural living are at natural food stores.

is, "absolutely!" Great care has been put into the development of these cleaning agents to ensure they work effectively in a wide variety of situations. On rare occasion a harsh chemical product may be required for a stubborn issue. However, using natural cleaning products is far more rewarding because the area doesn't stink of chemicals and synthetic perfumes after cleaning, but rather smells of citrus or other delightful plant or flower aromas. For example, I use Bi-O-Kleen laundry detergent, and I love the grapefruit fragrance of my freshly washed clothes.

Books & Resources
Natural food stores carry books and resources devoted to the natural living lifestyle. Some even have computers set up so you can look up a specific ailment or a natural healing remedy for further study. Because the store is devoted to natural living, some of the best books available on the subject will be on their shelves. You can find books about alternative therapies for specific ailments, vegetarian cooking, activism, parenting, yoga, and more.

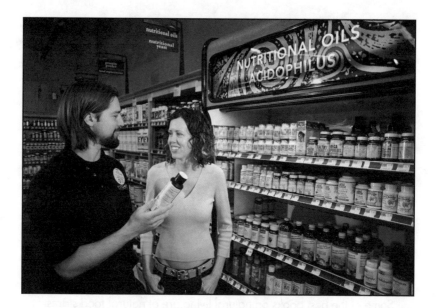

Knowledgeable Staff

You'll find that the natural food store staff members want to help you make the transition into the natural living lifestyle. Staff members at natural food stores usually have embraced the natural living lifestyle and are therefore friendly and enjoy helping their customers learn what they need to know on the path to natural living.

Classes & Workshops

Most of the larger natural food stores offer a variety of cooking classes as well as seminars on health issues, supplements and alternative therapies. Sometimes well-known authors speak or give workshops. Take advantage of these classes. You'll benefit from the support of the instructors and your classmates. What a great way to make new friends and get a jump start into the natural living lifestyle!

5
Healthy Eating
Follow the Essentials

There are many eating and dieting philosophies on the market to-day: they tell us to consume more protein and fewer carbohydrates, count our calories, eat certain fat-to-carbohydrate-to-protein ratios, or even to eat certain foods based on our blood type. Yet, eating for vibrant health does *not* need to be that complicated. The solution is simple: eat whole, fresh, raw and unprocessed foods, *as nature intended.* The majority of health problems plaguing most Americans today—degenerative dis-ease, obesity and low energy for starters—is primarily due to the national habit of eating over-processed, devitalized, pre-packaged, slightly toxic foods on a daily, weekly, monthly and yearly basis. It all adds up: *we are what we eat!*

In order to achieve optimal health, your goal is to eat a *variety* of fresh, whole, *organic,* nutrient-dense vegetables, fruits, grains, nuts, beans and legumes; and to eat only *organic* meat, if you eat meat. The organic produce section of your grocery store is your best friend. "Fresh, fresh, fresh—and organic" is your motto when shopping for food!

In our culture most of us constantly feel pressed for time, therefore we believe it takes too much time to prepare nutritious meals every day. We want convenience, so we buy prepackaged, canned or frozen foods. We are more than encouraged to choose this option by television, radio and print advertising and by the plethora of fast-food joints and junk food products that are readily available wherever we go. But these cul-

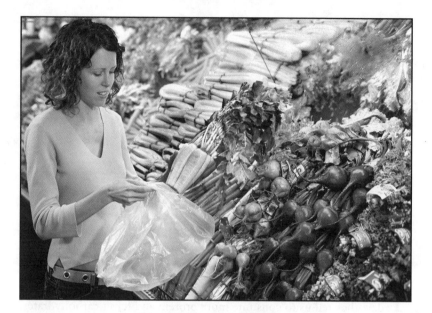

Eat fresh, raw, organic produce every day.

turally-sanctioned habits can literally *destroy our health*. Fortunately, the solution, unlike many diet programs, is not complicated.

Whole & Alive Food

There are two important components present in whole, raw foods that are critical to optimal health: 1) natural digestive enzymes and 2) the electromagnetic life force that flows through all living things (in Oriental medicine this is referred to as "chi" or "qi"). You'll learn more about the importance of chi in Chapter 9. Natural *digestive* enzymes are critical for good health and are found *only* in raw, whole plant foods. These important enzymes predigest our food and aid greatly in the absorption of nutrients. They are destroyed by cooking and industrial processing. Without them, only partial digestion occurs, placing a burden on the rest of the digestion process. An in-depth explanation of enzymes and their importance to our health is provided in the Supplements chapter.

As you might guess at this point, packaged, canned and frozen foods do not contain the live enzymes or chi that is present in fresh, organic foods. It is the "aliveness"—this electromagnetic life force—in *fresh produce* that we need for vibrant health! It is this same life force that pulses through our bodies and gives us our energy. Virtually *all* packaged foods are devoid of this life force. It's not present in animal foods. Cooking and freezing subdues it. Pasteurization deliberately destroys it. Thus, even most naturally processed food is usually devoid of the original life force. Eating a variety of raw (organic) plant food every day is extremely important for good health, and *far outweighs the benefits of any other dieting program.*

Packaged Foods
Should you shun all packaged foods in order to maintain health? Absolutely not. But packaged foods ought to be a *small* portion of your diet, not the majority of it. Why use frozen or canned vegetables when you can use fresh, organic vegetables? Perhaps the fresh version is out of season, you say. In that case, don't buy the canned or frozen version; instead, buy a different vegetable—one that is available in its raw, fresh form. If you know that certain produce is in season in your area, buy it instead of whatever has been shipped halfway around the world to your market. Buying local keeps money in your community, lowers pollution created by transporting non-local foods and provides you with what nature intends for you to eat during each season.

My general guideline regarding packaged food is to use canned, boxed (including bulk) or frozen food only if:

• It doesn't come fresh from the store (grains, beans, legumes, nuts, etc.), and
• It is going to be a small part of the larger meal, but *rarely* a meal unto itself.

Although I do eat pre-packaged meals on occasion (particularly Trader Joe's organic, frozen, vegetarian burritos), I don't make a habit of it. For example, instead of buying a can of chili, I'll buy a can of organic chili beans and then add fresh veggies, sautéed tempeh, spices and tamari (soy) sauce to make my own chili. My version is easy to prepare, tastes better, and is far more nutritious! My personal shopping list and quick-to-prepare meal suggestions are included in the Appendix to help give you a "jump start" as you explore this type of eating.

Acid/Alkaline Balance

Understanding the acid/alkaline balance is another key to achieving optimal health. Some foods cause the body's chemistry to be more acidic, while others cause it to be more alkaline. I'm not referring to stomach acid, but to the blood's pH and to the state of the fluids between our cells, which is called *intercellular* (or *interstitial) fluid*. An overly acidic condition (caused by eating too many acid-forming foods, by over-exercising or by habitually entertaining intense, negative emotions) forces the body to borrow minerals, including calcium, sodium, potassium and magnesium, from organs and bones to buffer (neutralize) the acid and safely remove it from the body.

Many experts in the alternative health field believe chronic acidity to be a *primary cause* of degenerative disease, because an acidic state allows pathogens to thrive, whereas an alkaline state does not. An acidic condition can cause severe damage to the body, which may go undetected for years. The kidneys are particularly susceptible because they flush out excess acid and must work much harder when such an "environment" is sustained. So our goal is to keep our bodily fluids more alkaline by eating alkaline-forming foods.

Processed foods (breads, pasta, cereals, coffee, sugar, white rice, boxed and canned foods), along with meat and dairy foods, contribute to an acidic state, whereas most whole, raw (unprocessed) organic plant foods contribute to an alkaline state. Although some raw foods are more acid forming than others, if you significantly limit meat, dairy and processed foods of all kinds, your acid/alkaline balance should be just fine. For more information, read the excellent book *Alkalize or Die*, by Theodore A. Baroody.

Yin/Yang Balance

The counterpart of the Western concept of the acid/alkaline balance is known in the Orient as the yin/yang principle. Yin is an expanding, feminine quality and yang is its complement: a contracting, masculine quality. Whereas the acid/alkaline balance is bio-chemically measurable, the yin/yang polarity is less concretely defined and is based on an electromagnetic energy model. Nevertheless, food (and everything else in existence) falls somewhere within this spectrum. And, like everything else, foods aren't purely yin or yang, but can be seen as containing more or less of

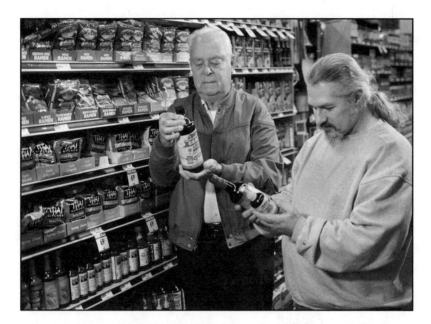

Braggs Liquid Aminos and shoyu sauce, found in the Macrobiotic section, are excellent salt replacers. I discuss them in the Appendix.

each quality in relation to or in comparison with other foods. For example, meat is considered to be very yang (grounding, contracting), and ice cream (especially because of the sugar it contains) is considered to be very yin (airy, expanding).

A predominance of either too much yin or too much yang energy not only throws our physiology out of balance, but also creates unbalanced states of consciousness. Have you ever talked with someone who seemed "spacey" to you? Perhaps s/he had trouble completing a sentence or fully explaining a thought or an idea before skipping to another, and another. That would be considered an *overly* yin (expanded consciousness) condition. On the other hand, you may know someone who has inflexible opinions, can't incorporate new ideas, may be loud and boisterous and doesn't want to listen to others. That is an *overly* yang (contracted consciousness) condition. The goal is to find ourselves balanced physically, mentally and emotionally between the two states, or just slightly more yang (grounded, but not overbearing and inflexible).

The Japanese macrobiotic philosophy incorporates the yin/yang principle and applies it to food very specifically. Thus, what we eat plays a *major role* in how yin or how yang we are (see chart).

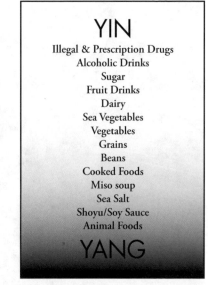

Overly yin conditions are usually caused by sweet foods and sugar, while overly yang conditions are often caused by too much meat and salt. Eating foods containing processed sugar (e.g. soda pop, candy, desserts, etc.) can create an extremely yin (expanded/"spaced out") state. Children who eat a lot of these foods (especially sugared cereal in the morning and soda in the afternoon) often have trouble concentrating in school. On the other hand, meat is extremely yang (grounding/contracting); therefore over-consumption of meat can cause aggression and inflexible attitudes. One reason why dessert is desired *after* a meat-based meal is to counter-balance the yang effects of the meat. Pretty interesting!

The effects of each food will be different for different people as well. A person whose constitution is more yin than yang may be thrown off balance by eating ice cream, while someone with a generally yang constitution may enjoy the same dessert without experiencing any imbalance. It's a complex, ever-changing dance of one element flowing into the other, but eating closer to the middle of the food spectrum (avoiding extremes) is wise. Limiting your intake of meat and *eliminating* sugary foods/candies/soda, as well as processed foods, is your best bet to developing yin/yang harmony.

Try to make food choices with the yin/yang balance in mind. Although you may desire to explore macrobiotic eating more closely, the most important thing to do is to avoid the extremes: sugary foods and too much meat. If you eat a variety of raw and cooked plant-based foods (cooking makes the food more yang), avoid sugar and refined foods and use tamari and sea salt for seasoning, you should stay well-balanced. For a deeper understanding of the yin/yang principles and macrobiotic cooking, read Herman Aihara's excellent book, *Basic Macrobiotics*, which can be found on Amazon.com (since it's no longer in print).

For vegetarians, who tend to be more yin because they aren't eating meat, I recommend making meals more yang by cooking part of the meal in tamari sauce (e.g., rice, beans, tempeh, veggies, etc.). Cooking makes the food more grounding, as does the tamari. Sea salt has the same effect. The one thing I find missing in most vegetarian philosophies is this crucial understanding of the yin/yang balance. The reason behind those "spacey" vegetarians is *not* a lack of protein, but rather a lack of yang energy.

Vegetarianism

A vegetarian shuns eating meat, but may eat eggs, fish and dairy. A vegan vegetarian (pronounced "vee-gan") avoids eating all animal or fish products. I began eating a vegan diet in 1990. After I adopted this lifestyle, I lost about 30 pounds, had more energy, didn't get sick as often and found that my mood was more consistently balanced and optimistic. Fourteen years later I still eat predominately a vegan diet, except for salmon every now and then. Many people assume it's difficult for me to eat this way, but as is the case with adopting any habit, I have found it to be fairly easy.

There are many sound nutritional and environmental reasons to eat a plant-based diet. The human digestive system is created to easily digest plant food, but not flesh, which makes us herbivores by nature. Consider that the hydrochloric acid in the human stomach is only 1/20th the strength of that found in carnivores. Carnivores require the stronger acid to process the flesh they consume. Human hydrochloric acid is designed for plant food, which means it can't fully process flesh. Furthermore, our intestines are 12 times the length of our body, whereas carnivores have intestines three times the length of their body. This is important because once a carnivore digests its prey, the remains needs to be quickly flushed through to prevent putrification (rotting). On the other hand, when humans eat meat, the combination of weak stomach acid and long intestines means putrification occurs throughout the digestive system, which can, and often does, lead to disease. Plant food, however, requires the longer journey to properly break down the fats, proteins, complex carbohydrates and nutrients.

The meat and dairy industry would have us believe that we can't get all our nutrients from just plant foods. This is simply ridiculous—our bodies are *designed* for plant food! Eating a *variety* of *organic* plant food grown in *optimum soil conditions* gives us all the vitamins, minerals, fats, essential fatty acids and protein we need.

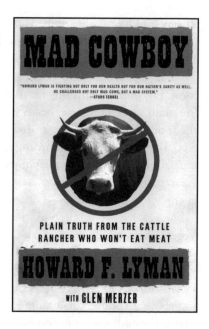

Non-organic meat may contain any number of contaminants, including multiple disease-causing organisms, high concentrations of pesticides and herbicides, tranquilizers, preservatives, artificial growth hormones, and the rendered parts of other diseased or dying animals. These contaminants contribute to a wide variety of diseases found in Americans today. And meat and dairy in general contribute to weight gain.

Mr. Lyman exposes the dark side of the meat and dairy industry.

Raising animals for food takes a huge toll on our water supply, as the following stunning statistics will illustrate. Over half of all the water used in the United States is for animal production. The water required to produce *five one-pound hamburgers* is equivalent to the amount of water a single-person household will use in a year! On the other hand, it only takes 25 gallons of water to produce one pound of wheat.

To make matters worse, the animal industry in the United States produces 130 times more excrement than humans do, and is the single largest source of water pollution in the U.S. What's worse is that virtually none of this excrement gets treated, and instead winds up polluting our water supply—decimating fish populations and aquatic life in the process.

Raising animals for food is also the single greatest reason for deforestation throughout our planet. For *every acre* of American forest that is cleared to make room for parking lots, roads, houses, shopping centers, etc., *seven acres* of forest is converted into land for grazing livestock

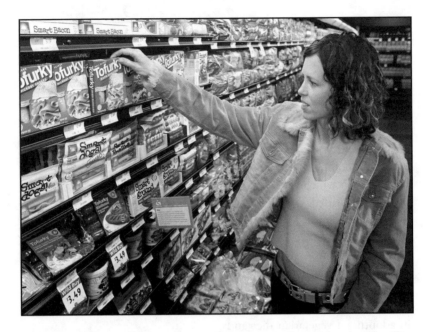

A wide variety of delicious meat substitutes—including products made from tempeh, tofu and seitan—are available at natural food stores.

and/or growing livestock feed. Every single day—worldwide—tropical rainforest about the size of New York City is decimated...forever. Most fast food chains get their beef from Central America, and the Rainforest Action Network (www.ran.org) estimates that about 55 square feet of tropical rainforest is required to produce just one hamburger.

Our demand for meat is so great that *virtually all animals* used for food today are grown in "factory farms." The problem with factory farms is that the animals—pigs and chickens—live in highly confined cages their entire lives, or, in the case of cows, live in cramped feedlots during the later part of their lives. They are fed scandalously substandard "food" such as their own excrement or rendered animals (including diseased and dying animals as well as deceased pets from veterinarians), and often go insane from their confinement.

Sickness is so rampant that animals must be given an assortment of drugs and antibiotics just to keep them alive long enough to get them to the slaughterhouse. Since profit is based on the weight of the animal, all sorts of cruel and unusual practices are used to make the animals gain weight unnaturally. Any person with ordinary sensibilities would find the conditions of any factory farm heartbreakingly cruel and abhorrent. But, out of sight, out of mind—you would never know by looking at the cheerful packaging in which the dead animals are presented.

If you eat meat, I strongly encourage you to switch to organic meat. This meat is by far much safer, and from what I've heard, much better tasting, than conventional meat. If you are interested in adopting a vegetarian diet and would like more information, I recommend reading the best book available on the subject: *The Food Revolution—How Your Diet Can Help Save Your Life and the World,* by John Robbins. Your life will be forever changed for the better when you read this excellent book.

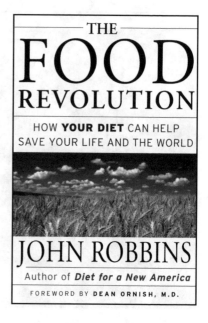

Mr. Robbins shatters the myth that we *must* eat meat for nutrition.

If you're going to eat a plant-based diet, the trick is to eat a variety of organic foods—grains, legumes, nuts, vegetables and fruits. What you don't want to do is eat processed foods or limit the types of plants you eat. Rather, mix it up and be adventurous. Plenty of examples are provided in the meal plans listed at the end of the book.

Dairy Products

Why are so many children allergic to cow's milk? Because they don't need it—not because there is something wrong with them. The revered pediatrician Benjamin Spock warned that "cow's milk…has definite faults for some babies. It causes allergies, indigestion, and contributes to some cases of childhood diabetes." Frank A. Oski, former director of pediatrics at Johns Hopkins University, bluntly stated: "There's no reason to drink cow's milk *at any time in your life*. It was designed for calves, not humans, and we should all stop drinking it today" (italics mine).

The intestines of some babies wind up bleeding after cow's milk has been consumed, resulting in iron loss. After age four, many children become lactose intolerant. For these children, milk proteins seep into the immune system and can result in chronic runny noses, sore throats, hoarseness, bronchitis, and recurring ear infections—the symptoms of "milk allergies." Some children's bodies react to cow's milk protein as a foreign substance, then produce high levels of antibodies in fending it off. These antibodies also destroy the cells that produce insulin in the pancreas, possibly paving the path toward diabetes.

Human breast milk is approximately five and a half percent protein, designed to double an infant's birth weight in about 180 days. Cow's milk, on the other hand, is about *fifteen* percent protein—it's meant to double the weight of a calf in just forty-seven days. Human babies who are fed cow's milk may only digest about half of the protein, straining their developing kidneys. When cow's milk mixes with an infant's digestive juices in the stomach, large curds develop because of the casein content, and that can lead to health problems. Whereas human milk is sterile, cow's milk is not, and feeding it to infants can introduce harmful organisms to a weak immune system. There's more saturated fat as well, which increases cholesterol in the infant. Pasteurization of cow's milk kills some harmful microorganisms, but it also destroys important lactobacillus bacteria and vitamins, which are normally found in human breast milk.

The high protein content of milk produces an acidic environment in the body. To correct the acidic environment, the body will withdraw calcium from the bones—which are alkaline—to bring the PH level back in balance. Although dairy is high in calcium, it can't be fully assimilated because of the high phosphorous content—calcium absorption occurs when there is a low phosphorous to high calcium ratio. The excess calcium floating in the blood, from the bones and from the milk, is then filtered through the kidneys, precipitating kidney stones later in life.

In addition to these issues, we also get the chemical stew from the aggressive agricultural practices found in the dairy industry. Dairy cows are unnaturally kept pregnant 24/7 to produce twenty times their normal amount of milk. They are housed in unsanitary conditions (often on conveyer belts). This leads to disease of the udder and to the dairy cows in general (including bovine leukemia, found in eighty-nine percent of dairy cows). Under these conditions, a cow's average lifespan drops from twenty years to about four. Antibiotics are used to slow disease, tranquilizers are used to calm frayed nerves, and artificial growth hormones are injected to increase milk production. The cows' feed is laden with pesticide and herbicide residue and other chemicals. Remember—what cows consume, we consume too.

Summary

For most of us, obesity, low energy, mood swings and health problems are associated with improper diet and can be corrected by changing what we eat and by following the other principles outlined in this book. When the body no longer takes in minute amounts of toxic chemicals and food additives every day, and instead receives bountiful nutrition, it begins to repair itself, shed pounds and move into balance. A balanced body contributes to a wonderful, deep-seated feeling of well-being that is not easily shaken by outside circumstances. All you need to know is that the true secret to eating properly is to avoid the foods discussed in Chapter 2 and to eat a wide *variety* of nutrient-dense *organic* plant food. By following this plan, you'll get all the calories, fats, proteins and carbohydrates you need, in the correct proportions.

Overview

1. Eat a *variety* of whole, raw, organic plant foods (fruits, veggies, grains, legumes, beans and nuts).
2. If you eat meat, eat only organic meat, and avoid dairy products.
3. Use pre-packaged foods sparingly (boxed, canned, frozen).
4. Minimize acid-forming foods (meats, packaged/processed foods).
5. Maximize alkaline forming foods (organic plant foods).
6. Avoid extremely yin foods (soda pop, sugary foods, candies, etc.)
7. Minimize extremely yang foods (meats: beef, pork and chicken).
8. Use sea salt instead of iodized salt. Don't use hydrogenated oils.
9. If vegetarian, use shoyu or tamari sauce and cook some of your food (for grounded energy).
10. Follow my personal shopping list and meal suggestions in the Appendix and you'll get the hang of it in no time!

6
Supplements
Use Often for Health

Most soil is depleted of many important minerals, which means that our food—even organic food—doesn't always have optimum nutritional value. One of the best ways to overcome this deficiency is to take supplements on a regular basis.

There are hundreds of supplements to choose from, which can make it pretty confusing to choose which are best for you. In this chapter I cover some of the more common supplements you may want to take on a daily basis. Whenever possible, use "whole food" supplements; these contain most or all of the original components of the source from which the supplement was derived. Often, they are very "nutrient-dense," the way nature intended.

Green Superfoods
Most natural food stores sport a "green foods" section, which makes it easy to find this type of supplement. You'll find products such as alfalfa, barley grass, chlorella, spirulina and wild blue-green algae, as well as custom blends that contain many or all of these plants and algae. Besides offering a variety of minerals, vitamins, amino acids and essential fatty acids, they all contain chlorophyll—a unique and important blood builder. I'll discuss the properties of chlorophyll first, then the benefits of drinking live wheat grass juice, and then get into some of the specific superfoods you can find in that "green" section of the supplement aisle.

Chlorophyll

Chlorophyll is the molecule that absorbs sunlight and uses its energy to synthesize carbohydrates from carbon dioxide and water. Known as photosynthesis, this is the basis for sustaining the life processes of all plants. Since animals and humans obtain their food supply by eating plants, photosynthesis can be said to be the source of our life also.

Interestingly, the molecular structure of chlorophyll is remarkably similar to that of hemoglobin, which is found in red blood cells. The main difference is that the central atom in chlorophyll is magnesium, whereas in hemoglobin it's iron. Hemoglobin has a strong iron bond, and chlorophyll has a weak magnesium bond. In the human body chlorophyll releases the magnesium bond and a cellular vortex starts sucking in heavy metals and cleansing the blood. Thus, chlorophyll is considered a major blood purifier, and is very beneficial for overall health.

According to Paul Pitchford, author of *Healing with Whole Foods*, chlorophyll provides numerous health benefits. It stops bacterial growth in wounds, eliminates bad breath and body odor, removes drug deposits, and counteracts all toxins, including radiation. It also builds blood, renews tissue, promotes healthful intestinal flora, activates enzymes that produce vitamins A, D, and K, reverses anemic conditions, reduces high blood pressure, strengthens the immune system, relieves nervousness and serves as a mild diuretic.[1] All of the following green products contain high amounts of chlorophyll (some more than others) to give you the benefit of its highly rejuvenating effects.

Wheat Grass Juice

"Fifteen pounds of wheat grass is equal in overall nutritional value to 350 pounds of ordinary garden vegetables. We have not even scratched the surface of what grass can mean to man in the future."[2]
—Dr. Charles Schnabel, Father of Wheat Grass Therapy

In 1930, American Dr. Charles Franklin Schnabel—whose background was in agricultural chemistry and soil fertility—discovered that feeding fresh oat grass to 108 hens helped them overcome disease. Soon afterward they doubled their egg production. Dr. Schnabel's interest was so piqued by this discovery that he began a quest to find out if fresh grass from grains could improve the health of other animals, or of humans. For years he fed the fresh grass to both animals and humans, and had the grass analyzed at laboratories. He discovered that grass from grains, especially barley and wheat, was packed with all the necessary nutrients required to survive, overcome disease and help attain vibrant health. By 1940, Dr. Schnabel's research proved to be so valuable to the health of Americans that cans of his grass were for sale in major drug stores throughout the United States and Canada.

Unfortunately, World War II changed that. After the end of the war, large corporations influenced American eating habits and medical choices towards chemicals and drugs, and the companies Dr. Schnabel was associated with discontinued distribution of his grass products. By 1950, Americans had been shifted from a natural to a synthetic approach to health care, and it wouldn't be until the 1970s that natural grasses would make a comeback, largely due to a few committed individuals. Today you can find fresh wheat grass juice in most natural foods stores and juice bars because of those pioneers, and for good reason.

Grass from grains such as barley, wheat, oat, kamut and rye—when harvested just before they produce a grain—are a powerhouse of nutrition. Think of how massive cows, antelope, deer, bison, elephants and many other animals become—just from eating grass! That's because grass has all the major and trace minerals we require, are packed full of vitamins (including all the Bs—even B-12), have all the essential amino acids, contain essential fatty acids and contain over 80 enzymes. They also provide protein in the form of poly-peptides, which are assimilated faster than meat-based protein, and are very abundant in chlorophyll.

For health maintenance, 1 to 2 ounces of wheat grass juice (often taken in "shots") is plenty; four or more ounces a day is recommended during cleansing and/or for overcoming health challenges. The sweetness of the juice is part of its power—the sugar in the grass helps deliver the chlorophyll into the bloodstream quickly. The sugars crystallize in the intestinal tract, which draws toxins out of the tissues. One ounce of wheat grass juice can contain up to 18,000 units of beta-carotene (precursor of vitamin A, an immune builder), has abundant vitamin E (which fights cancer growth) and a large amount of vitamin K (for proper blood clotting). The juice is loaded with enzymes that help detoxify harmful substances and that participate in thousands of the constant chemical changes taking place in the body.

Although it is a nutritional powerhouse, the most unique aspect of fresh wheat grass juice is probably its "aliveness." This "liquid sunshine" abounds with an electromagnetic life force (sometimes referred to as "prana," "chi" or "qi" energy, see Chapter 9). When the concentrated energy of wheat grass enters the body, it has a profound healing effect on everything it contacts. Freshly picked vegetables, especially leafy greens, have this energy as well, but it's so concentrated in fresh wheat grass juice that you can feel it as soon as you drink it.

In his book, *Wheat Grass—Nature's Finest Food,* Steve Meyerowitz documents dozens of people's stories about the healing effects of using fresh wheat grass juice as an adjunct to their healing process. Real-life stories of people overcoming breast, bladder, prostate, colon, throat, lymph and liver cancers, as well as candidiasis, irritable bowel and leaky gut syndromes, lyme disease, lupus and more are documented in his book.

Generally, wheat grass juice is taken on an empty stomach at least half an hour before a meal. You can find it at your local juice bar or natural food store, or buy a wheat grass juicer (different from a vegetable juicer) for around $200 and juice wheat grass at home. Purveyors of wheat grass juice can usually sell you trays of the grass for home juicing as well. Everything in my book is important, but drinking wheat grass juice on a regular basis, in my opinion, is one of the most important things you can do for your health.

Alfalfa

Taken as a liquid extract, alfalfa has a rich mineral profile and contains abundant chlorophyll. Alfalfa roots can dig down over 100 feet, giving the plant access to minerals and trace minerals that other plants can't acquire.

The Arabs were the first to name alfalfa, which means "father of all foods."[3] Alfalfa cleans and tones the intestines and removes harmful acids from the blood. Alfalfa is rich in protein, carotene, calcium, iron, magnesium, potassium, phosphorus, sodium, sulfur, silicon, cobalt and zinc. Alfalfa provides these minerals in a balanced form, which promotes absorption. Alfalfa also contains eight enzymes that help assimilate protein, fats and carbohydrates. Alfalfa alkalizes and detoxifies the body, especially the liver.

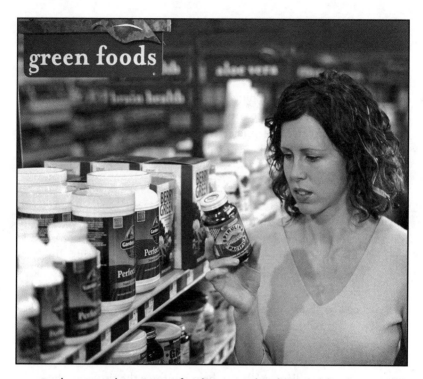

Find nutrient dense green foods at your local natural food store.

Barley Grass

Barley is an annual cereal plant that has been cultivated for hundreds of years. Although the barley grain is most often used, the plant's true nutrition is found in the leaves—the young green shoots that form before the grain sprouts. This green grass is reputed to be the only vegetation on earth that could supply our sole nutritional support from birth to old age!

Barley grass contains an astounding amount of vitamins and minerals, including five of the B vitamins (the often hard to obtain B12 being among them). It also contains folic acid, pantothenic acid, beta carotene, C and E. Recent laboratory analysis on green barley grass has turned up traces of more than 70 minerals, among them calcium, iron, magnesium, and phosphorus (which is determined, in part, by soil conditions).

Barley grass also contains 18 amino acids, which are the building blocks of proteins. Green barley grass is also said to have a highly alkalizing effect, because it contains buffering minerals such as sodium, potassium, calcium and magnesium.

Micro-Algae

Spirulina, chlorella and wild blue-green algae are the most common commercial micro-algae. All three contain the highest sources of chlorophyll, protein, beta-carotene and nucleic acids of any animal or plant food, making them some of the best possible supplements you can take on a regular basis.

Spirulina

Spirulina is a naturally digestible food that helps to protect the immune system, lower cholesterol and facilitate mineral absorption. Spirulina is high in chlorophyll, protein, beta-carotene and nucleic acids. Interestingly, the protein digestibility of spirulina is rated at 85%, versus about 20% for beef.[4]

The cell wall of spirulina is composed entirely of mucopolysaccharides (MPs), which are complex sugars interlaced with amino acids, simple sugars and sometimes protein. MPs are fully digestible and help strengthen body tissues, especially the connective tissues, making them more elastic and resilient. MPs also help reinforce the tissues of the heart and guard against deterioration of the arteries.

Spirulina is packed with other nutrients, including vitamin B12, one that many believe is only available from animal foods (although some scientists dispute just how bio-available the B12 is in spirulina). It has a rich supply of the blue pigment phycocyanin, a light-harvesting pigment that has been shown to inhibit the development of cancer.

This amazing whole food detoxifies the liver and kidneys, builds and enriches the blood, cleanses the arteries, enhances intestinal flora, and inhibits the growth of fungi, bacteria, and various strains of yeast. A number of manufacturers make it available as a powder, capsule or tablet, and you may want to buy it less expensively in the bulk section. Just stir a heaping teaspoonful into your favorite juice drink.

Chlorella

Chlorella contains 10 to 100 times more chlorophyll than leafy green vegetables. Chlorella is grown in controlled mediums where minerals are added to optimize it for human consumption. Its small size requires centrifuge harvesting and special processing to improve the digestibility of the tough outer wall, which makes it more expensive than spirulina. However, the cell wall binds to heavy metals, pesticides and carcinogens such as PCBs and escorts the toxins out of the body, making it a particularly valuable supplement.

Chlorella has less protein and a fraction of the beta-carotene than spirulina, but more than twice the nucleic acid and chlorophyll. Nucleic acid (RNA/DNA) in the body is responsible for cell renewal, growth and repair. Insufficient nucleic acid causes premature aging and a weakened immune system. Chlorella is also abundant in iron, zinc and vitamin A, which helps boost the immune system.

Wild Blue-Green Algae (*Aphanizomenon flos-acquae*)
Whereas spirulina and chlorella are grown in man-made tanks, wild blue-green algae grows naturally in Upper Klamath Lake in Southern Oregon, making it a particularly unique whole food supplement. This single-celled micro-algae was first discovered over 15 years ago in one of the most diverse and rich wetland habitats in North America. It is harvested at the peak of its bloom in summer, and then quickly freeze-dried to preserve its nutritional profile and enzymatic activity.

Upper Klamath Lake has an average depth of about eight feet, yet the algae feeds on mineral rich sediment that is believed to be at least 35 feet deep. It's estimated that just one inch of this mineral rich sediment, generated over 10,000 years ago from a volcanic explosion, is able to produce enough algae to feed every person on the planet one gram a day for the next sixty years!

Many believe it is the "wild" nature of blue-green algae that gives it such an excellent nutritional profile. The chlorophyll content is twice as high as that of spirulina.

Aphanizomenon flos-acquae (AFA) is a nutritional powerhouse. Over 98% of its nutrients are bio-available, which means they can be used directly by the body in the same form in which they naturally occur. Amino acids are the building blocks of proteins (and muscle tissue), and AFA contains all eight essential amino acids, in the correct profile for optimum absorption. AFA contains up to 68% more protein by weight than any other whole food. It also has high neuropeptide concentrations to help repair, rebuild and strengthen neurotransmitters in the brain so that neurons can communicate optimally with the rest of the body. Nearly 50% of AFA's lipid content is the essential fatty acid alpha-linolenic acid (omega-3). Omega-3 fatty acids support the immune system and build the white fatty myelin sheath on connective neural fibers in the brain. People who eat AFA on a regular basis report an overall increase in mental alertness and stamina, improved short and long-term memory, enhanced creativity and problem-solving abilities, as well as a greater sense of well being.

AFA has a full spectrum of naturally chelated minerals and trace minerals, as well as a wide range of vitamins. One gram of wild blue-green algae supplies 48% of the recommended daily requirement of Vitamin B1 (beta-carotene), 133% of Vitamin B12 and significant amounts of all the B complex vitamins. The protein rich cell wall of AFA is a source of glycogen, used by the liver for energy, which is one reason people often report an increase in energy after adding it to their daily diet.

Probiotics (Friendly Microflora)
"Probiotic," literally meaning "for life," is a term used to describe the friendly bacteria and fungi which inhabit both the large and small intestines. There are at least 400 different species of micro-flora that live in the human gastrointestinal tract. There are billions of these microbes, amounting to approximately three pounds per adult! Some of the most important of these bacteria are acidophilus (*Lactobacillus acidophilus)*, which inhabit the small intestine and bifidus (*Bifidobacterium bifidum*), which inhabit the large intestine.

All of our organs are important, but as you'll learn in the detoxification section, the colon requires your attention first, because when it doesn't function properly, it affects the ability of all other organs to function optimally. I suggest taking daily supplements of acidophilis and bifidus because they are easily destroyed by factors such as antibiotics, stress, alcohol, high meat/fat diets, drugs and poor diet in general.

The small intestine is involved in the digestion, absorption, and transport of food. After passing through the stomach, food is further broken down in the small intestine; and vitamins, minerals, carbohydrates, protein, and fat are absorbed. Microvilli—hair-like projections along the wall of the small intestine—perform two important functions: they provide necessary surface area for the absorption of nutrients and they help move food through the small intestine. Acidophilus helps to keep the spaces between the microvilli clear so they can function efficiently. Thus, acidophilus helps to promote normal peristalsis (movement of food) through the small intestine.

Acidophilus plays a role in the prevention of and defense against disease, especially of the gastrointestinal tract and vagina. As part of the "normal flora," they inhibit the growth of harmful organisms by competing for nutrients, altering the pH to a more acidic level, and shifting oxygen levels to the detriment of pathogens (disease- causing organisms). They also attach to sites otherwise preyed upon by pathogens.

Other benefits of acidophilus include: production of vitamins (which are absorbed into the blood); the synthesis of many B vitamins, including biotin and folic acid; an increase in the absorption of calcium, phosphorus and magnesium; normalization of cholesterol levels in the blood and production of digestive enzymes. Acidophilus also helps maintain bowel regularity. Acidophilus supplements have been shown to help reduce or eliminate intestinal, vaginal and urinary tract infections. Because this friendly bacteria promotes healthy intestinal functioning, it has been found to be useful in helping overcome many other diseases.[5]

Bifidus helps repopulate the large intestine with friendly bacteria, creating a favorable environment for large intestine health. Bifidus lowers the pH of the intestines, manufactures specific B vitamins, ensures regular bowel movements, and can help stop gas and bloating while promoting proper immune function and overall health. Finally, eating a diet rich in plant foods will help to naturally cultivate a healthy balance of probiotic organisms.

Enzymes

Enzymes are considered the "sparks of life." Even with appropriate levels of minerals, vitamins, amino acids, water and other nutrients, without enzymes, life ceases to exist. For this reason, they are said to possess life force energy. These energized protein molecules play a necessary role in virtually all biochemical activities. They are required to digest food and to repair cells, tissues and organs. In fact, they regulate and govern all living cells in plants and animals, and are responsible for providing the energy for all biochemical reactions that occur in nature. Fruit ripening, seeds sprouting, flowers blooming and people healing are all examples of enzymatic activity. Enzymes cannot be made from synthetic (non-plant) sources, as many vitamins and minerals are made.

Enzymes and coenzymes (molecules that help enzymes do their job) work together to either join molecules together or split them apart by making or breaking chemical bonds. Most enzymes are composed of a protein coupled with an essential mineral, and sometimes a vitamin, which act as the co-enzyme.

There are three major enzymatic classifications: metabolic, digestive and those obtained from food. Metabolic and digestive enzymes are produced in the body, but food enzymes are not—they only come from food. Processing or cooking food above 112 degrees destroys food enzymes.

"Metabolic enzymes" build the body from proteins, carbohydrates and fats, and break them apart when they are old. All our cells, tissues and organs function because of these enzymes. They are responsible for chemical reactions within cells, such as energy production and detoxification. Each body tissue/system produces its own specific set of metabolic enzymes. Metabolic enzymes cannot be supplied through supplementation.

"Digestive enzymes" are secreted along the gastrointestinal tract and help break down foods, enabling nutrients to be absorbed into the bloodstream. Our bodies manufacture and secrete about 24 different digestive enzymes depending on the type of food we eat. Digestive enzymes break down food particles for storage in the liver or in muscles. This stored energy is later converted by other enzymes for use by the body when needed.

"Food enzymes" come from plants, and are vulnerable to processing and temperatures above 112 degrees. These vital helpers predigest our food and aid greatly in the absorption of nutrients. Without them (either from food or supplementation), the natural process of full digestion is lost, which puts an undue strain on the digestive system.

The three major food enzymes are: amylase, which breaks down starches into sugars; lipase, which breaks down fats into fatty acids, and protease, which breaks down proteins into amino acids. Protease is also used therapeutically for digesting viruses and bacteria, and for eliminating allergies.

Enzymes can be found in many different plant foods, but the plant must be fresh and whole in order to contain live enzymes (unless it's been specifically processed to retain the enzymes). Some foods that contain lots of enzymes include avocados, papayas, pineapples, bananas and mangos. Sprouts are one of the richest sources of enzymes. Many companies process these foods into enzyme supplements. Many pickled (or fermented) foods, as well as miso paste, also contain enzymes. Unless at least 50% of your diet consists of organic, whole, raw plant foods that contain naturally occurring food enzymes, you may want to take a daily enzyme supplement for better absorption of the food you eat.

Flaxseed Oil (For Omega-3/6 Essential Fatty Acids)
Flaxseed oil is one of the best sources for essential fatty acids, which are the basic building blocks of fats. Essential fatty acids are considered essential because they are needed for normal cell structure and function, yet our bodies do not manufacture them. They are categorized as omega-3 (n-3) and omega-6 (n-6) (the number describes the place of the first double bond in these poly-unsaturated fatty acids (PUFAs)) and are required for proper functioning of nerve cells and cell membrane walls.

All our cells are enveloped by a membrane composed mostly of essential fatty acid compounds called phospholipids, which play a major role in determining the integrity and fluidity of the membranes. The type of fat we consume determines the type of phospholipid in the cell membrane. Unfortunately, the Standard American Diet (S.A.D.) severely *lacks* essential fatty acids. *Instead,* it is high in animal fats, which are high in saturated fatty acids, cholesterol, and trans-fatty acids (also formed by chemical extraction or high-heat processing and hydrogenation of unsaturated plant oils), giving our cells the wrong ratio of fatty acids. This imbalance leads to cell membranes that contain less fluid, making it difficult for them to perform their primary function: acting as a selective barrier that regulates the passage of nutrients and wastes in and out of the cell.

Without a healthy membrane, cells lose vital nutrients, electrolytes and their ability to hold water. They also lose their ability to communicate efficiently with other cells and respond appropriately to regulating hormones. Diminished cellular function is one of the primary causes of degenerative disease. A diet high in animal foods, combined with improperly processed oils, puts us at great risk.

On the flip side, research has shown that diets high in omega-3 fatty acids help prevent heart attacks, lower blood pressure, reduce allergies and inflammation, relieve or reverse symptoms of multiple sclerosis, offer anti-cancer properties, and may help combat a host of degenerative diseases.[6] This is because the essential fatty acids 3 and 6 are also transformed into regulatory compounds known as prostaglandins. Prostaglandins regulate steroid production and hormone synthesis; they also regulate pressure in the eye, joints and blood vessels. Additionally, they mediate immune response, regulate bodily secretions and their viscosity, dilate or constrict blood vessels, regulate the rate at which cells divide and regulate the flow of substances in and out of cells. There's still more the busy prostaglandins do: they transport oxygen from red blood cells to bodily tissues, regulate nerve transmission and assist in other vital functions. As you can see, essential fatty acids are, well, *essential*, in our diet. Yet few of us get enough of them, because most of us don't eat foods high in essential fatty acids, and we do eat foods that diminish or neutralize them.

Omega-6 fatty acids can be found in raw nuts, seeds, and legumes, and in unsaturated (cold-pressed) vegetable oils such as flaxseed, borage, grape seed, primrose, sesame and soybean. Omega-3 fatty acids can be found in deepwater fish, fish oil and vegetable oils such as canola, walnut and flaxseed.[7] Based on my research, I believe that organic, expeller-pressed flaxseed oil is an excellent source of both omega-3 and omega-6 essential fatty acids. Flaxseed oil contains 58% omega-3 fatty acid, which is twice the amount found in fish oil, which may be contaminated by pesticide and/or chemical residue (such as mercury).

Two tablespoons of flaxseed oil a day seems to be the recommendation by most sources. I pour some on my morning miso soup (see the Appendix), and the nutty flavor of flax oil is also delicious on salads, baked foods such as potatoes, and on bread. You'll find it in the supplements/refrigerator section of the natural foods store. Check both the "pressing" and expiration dates to be sure the product is fresh.

Additional note: As explained in Chapter 2, I suggest avoiding all hydrogenated oils (margarine) as well any oil that is not organic and expeller-pressed. The best oils will be found in opaque bottles to reduce potential rancidity. The only company I'm aware of which has a full line of oils bottled in opaque containers is Omega Nutrition. The two best tasting flax seed oils are made by Omega Nutrition and Barlean's.

Apple Cider Vinegar

Pure, organic, uncooked and non-pasteurized apple cider vinegar is another indispensable item you'll want to have on hand. Although not a supplement per se, it offers multiple (and inexpensive) benefits. It is a natural antibiotic and antiseptic that fights germs, bacteria, mold and viruses.

Apple cider vinegar has been referred to as one of nature's most perfect foods. Made from fresh, crushed apples (look for those allowed to mature in wooden barrels, as wood seems to boost natural fermentation), apple cider vinegar (ACV) has a long, fascinating history. From the beginning of recorded history, all ancient civilizations have utilized vinegar (often with wine). Vinegar was used as a healing elixir by Hippocrates (the "Father of Medicine") and it has been found in Egyptian urns as far back as 3000 BCE. The Babylonians are said to have used it as a condiment and preservative, while the Greeks and Romans used it both for flavoring and healing purposes. Parisians used it in the Middle Ages as a deodorant and healing tonic—it was even touted as a preserver of youth! Columbus had vinegar barrels on his sailing vessels to prevent scurvy. Japanese Samurai warriors drank ACV for strength and power, and it was used during the Civil War to disinfect and heal wounds.

Modern day use includes spot and stain removal as well as color preservation. Save the popular white, distilled vinegar for carpets and the laundry. Our society has come to equate clear/white products with purity and cleanliness, yet often that means toxic bleach and byproducts. In the case of distilled white vinegar, powerful enzymes, trace minerals and natural malic and tartaric acids (which fight toxins and bacteria) are destroyed by heat during the distillation process. Distilled white vinegar also contains acetic acid, which is detrimental to the health of the body. This acid is known to rapidly destroy red blood cells, interfere with digestion and contribute to liver and intestinal problems.[8] You want undistilled, naturally fermented and organic ACV with a rich, brownish color. Don't be turned off by the "cobweb-like" substance you may see—those are important strands of protein molecules and pectin. This life- giving substance is called "the mother" by Paul Bragg, N.D.—one of America's original "health food" advocates. He and his daughter Patricia are authors of *Apple Cider Vinegar.*[9]

Also beware of "sanitized" ACVs and malt vinegars that lack the health giving properties of the real thing, and avoid imitations made (here's a designer food for you) from coal tar (the product, since it's cheaper than distilled or malt vinegar, is the most popular vinegar in supermarkets today).

As those sophisticated Middle Age Parisians knew, apples are a rich source of potassium, which is necessary for the soft tissues of the body, just like calcium is required for our bones. Potassium is the "mineral of youthfulness," keeping the arteries flexible and resilient. Potassium is also responsible for good skin and muscle tone. Before you turn to plastic surgery for drooping eyelids, reach for a bottle of apple cider vinegar. You may be suffering from a potassium deficiency, which can be easily and inexpensively corrected by a daily dose. Potassium helps give rigidity to plant stems and assists them to grow and blossom. When a plant suffers potassium deficiency, it yellows, withers and dies. Potassium makes the flesh of farm animals healthier and tender. The main function of potassium in people is to keep the tissues healthy, soft and pliable, and to help prevent heart attacks and strokes. Our bodies are meant to be self-cleansing, self-correcting, self-repairing and self-healing. With potassium—the master mineral—toxic poisons are literally placed "in solution" so they can be flushed out of the body.

A fresh, organically grown apple contains living enzymes, phosphorus, chlorine, potassium, sodium, magnesium, calcium, sulfur, iron, fluorine, silicon, along with vitamins and minerals, and over 10,000 micronutrients! It also contains oxygen, water, and many other important trace elements and compounds in the proper ratio for the body to use. The saying, "an apple a day keeps the doctor away" may well be true. There's usually little we can do to improve on nature, but fermenting those fresh apples seems to be an exception. ACV truly seems to be of benefit in almost any condition imaginable.

Even the healthiest of us needs to clear the body of "acid crystal" buildup, easily done by drinking a cocktail of distilled water, ACV and honey every day. Gabriel Cousens M.D., author of *Conscious Eating*, says "Organic apple cider vinegar is the #1 food I recommend for maintaining the body's vital acid/alkaline balance." The following list illustrates some of the other benefits of apple cider vinegar.

- Relieves dandruff, itchy scalp, thinning hair and even baldness (add royal jelly and leave on overnight)
- Soothes tired, aching muscles and joints (take a warm bath containing 1 cup ACV)
- Strengthens the heart and reduces arrhythmia
- Aids blood vessels, arteries and veins
- Improves digestion
- Relieves chronic fatigue
- Zaps sore throats and laryngitis (gargle)
- Treats insect bites
- Is an effective aid for female discomforts and can help shrink an enlarged prostate
- Helps control and normalize weight
- Helps lower blood pressure
- Eases arthritis (by flushing toxic crystals from joints)

You can also make hot & cold vinegar compresses or vaporize ACV to help relieve headaches. Apple cider vinegar supplies the eyes with needed tissue mineral salts, and two or three drops of a solution of ACV and water two to three times daily has been said to remove cataracts! Breathing the steamy vapors of heated ACV can clear nasal passages for 12 to 24 hours, while gargling with it can relieve sore throats. Sipping a mixture of ACV and water can relieve a tickling cough as well as relieve laryngitis and asthma. Sipping ACV with water every five minutes will help alleviate nausea, food poisoning and diarrhea, while a teaspoonful can eliminate hiccups. Swishing a mixture of ACV and water can eliminate "morning breath." As a mouthwash, it helps prevent tartar deposits. Brushing your teeth with the same solution will whiten them as well as protect them from decay. Applied to the skin it soothes sunburn and can relieve eczema and shingles.[10]

Whew! What a bang for your buck. I prefer Braggs Apple Cider Vinegar, found at all natural food stores. If drinking the liquid mixture doesn't appeal to you, most health food stores have ACV tablets. Each tablet is usually equivalent to one teaspoon (±) of ACV.

Antioxidants

Antioxidants are a group of chemicals that devour free radicals. Many of these antioxidants are phytochemicals (plant products) that are obtained by a diet rich in fruits and vegetables. However, there are animal antioxidants, such as Co-Q10, and minerals such as selenium, that act as antioxidants. Free radicals are created when cells are under attack from various toxins, viruses, germs or fungi. They are caused by tobacco smoke, pollution, stress, and hydrogenated, overheated or rancid oils; and they are almost always produced by fried foods.

If left unchecked, free radicals damage cells, leading to a suppressed immune system and, subsequently, to degenerative disease. They are a primary cause of wrinkles and sagging skin. Combat them with the high concentration of antioxidants found in wheat grass juice, barley grass, sprouts and dark green vegetables. For added protection, you may want to take a daily supplement. Three popular antioxidants found in natural foods stores are: coenzyme Q_{10} (Co-Q_{10}), grape seed extract and pycnogenol. The later two are oligomeric proanthocyanidins (OPCs), substances that are related to tannins and have benefits in addition to their antioxidant properties. Pycnogenol is a trade name for OPCs derived from a pine tree. Other supplements with antioxidant properties include the herbs bilberry and Ginkgo biloba, and green tea. And don't forget vitamins A, C, and E, all of which have important antioxidant functions.

Garlic

Garlic has been used since biblical times and has an amazing array of healing properties. It contains an amino acid derivative called alliin. When you eat garlic, the enzyme alliinase converts alliin into allicin, which has an antibiotic effect. Another component of garlic is methyl allyl trisulfide, which dilates blood vessel walls. Garlic also contains many sulfur compounds that promote healing.

Garlic is known to increase circulation; remove abdominal obstructions; eliminate parasites, yeast, worms and bad bacteria; relieve the stinging of insect bites, nettles, poison ivy and oak; clear ear infections; detoxify the body; enhance immune system function; lower blood pressure and help promote healing of virtually all diseases.

One drawback to garlic, according to some Oriental traditions, is that it can stimulate excessive emotional/sexual desire, an effect those on a spiritual path may want to avoid or minimize. Garlic can also thin the blood, so care must be taken if you are already on an anticoagulant. Garlic can be eaten raw, or taken as an encapsulated supplement. Cooked garlic does not retain the properties of raw and supplemental garlic.

Conclusion

For superior health, I suggest taking a whole green superfood (e.g., alfalfa, barley grass, chlorella, spirulina and/or AFA), probiotics, enzymes, antioxidants and flax seed oil every day. Add wheat grass juice and garlic every day if you are working to heal a condition, or on occasion if you are in fairly good health and have no specific health problems. If price is a factor and you can't afford everything I've listed, give probiotics (intestinal health) first priority, then flax oil, then bulk spirulina.

There are hundreds of other supplements available, but the ones listed above will give you a good start towards attaining and maintaining vibrant health. To learn more about nutritional supplements, I recommend the exceptionally well written and researched book, *Encyclopedia of Nutritional Supplements* by Michael T. Murray, N.D. Another awesome resource book is *Prescription for Nutritional Healing* by James Balch, M.D. and Phyllis Balch, C.N.C.

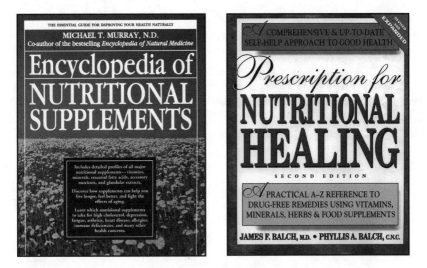

I highly recommend these two reference books.

7
Detoxification
Cleanse Yourself of Toxins

All of us take in minute amounts of poison every day. Much of the food we eat contains pesticides, herbicides, dyes, preservatives, flavorings, stabilizers, processing chemicals, artificial growth hormones, antibiotics and even tranquilizers (found in meat). On top of that, most conventionally packaged foods have been over-processed and therefore devitalized of innate nutritional value. When the body is *overloaded* with these poisons, the detoxifying organs, such as the liver, kidney and skin, are compromised. When this happens, the immune system is weakened, other systems don't function properly, and disease can occur. To prevent disease from gaining a foothold in your body, it is important to stop taking in toxins (as discussed in Chapter 2) and remove those already stored in your body (called detoxification).

If you truly want vibrant health, you can't neglect this step! If you are in poor health, have a medical condition or are taking prescription drugs, I strongly recommend that you visit a naturopathic doctor (discussed in Chapter 10) and request guidance on a detoxification program. Following the guidelines I outline in this chapter will be very beneficial, but a naturopathic doctor will be able to determine your toxicity level and the best methods for removing the toxins. Also, "detoxing" too quickly can flood your system and cause a "healing crisis." Slow down if you start having symptoms and, again, consider getting some professional guidance.

ise

Cl... it your colon (large intestine) is one of the most important things you can do to achieve vibrant health. It's not something I thought much about until I read *Cleanse & Purify Thyself,* by Dr. Richard Anderson, a book I highly recommend. What I learned is that the colon becomes quite clogged after years of poor eating. Once the buildup occurs, disease is almost sure to manifest.

According to Dr. Anderson, when we eat poorly on a continual basis (or the wrong foods on an occasional basis), the intestines react by secreting a protective mucoid layer to prevent the absorption of toxins. This protective mechanism

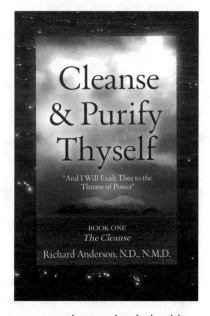

Dr. Anderson's book should be read by everyone.

was designed for the occasional ingestion of bad or rotten food, not for the daily abuse that the Standard American Diet (S.A.D.) places on our digestive system. When we eat incorrectly on occasion, the pancreatic juices will strip the mucoid layer off within a few days; but a daily barrage of over-processed and chemically laden foods creates a buildup of the stuff (called fecal mucoid matter), and that causes problems.

After years of eating a poor diet we will accumulate this mucoid matter (which often causes a bulging of the gut). As a result, food moves more slowly through the intestines, nutrients aren't well absorbed, moisture is decreased, worms and parasites colonize, unfriendly bacteria thrive, free radicals are formed, toxins can't be properly eliminated, and then various diseases of the intestine may appear. Fecal mucoid matter buildup results in fermentation, putrification (rotting) and stagnant pus pockets filled with various poisons and harmful bacteria (hence the foul smells when gas is passed). Or, disease can manifest anywhere in the body because, as Dr. Bernard Jensen says, "every tissue of the body is fed by the blood, which is supplied by the bowel. When the bowel is dirty, the blood is dirty, and so on to the organs and tissues. *It is the bowel that invariably has to be cared for before any effective healing can take place.*[1] (Italics mine.) One major problem with a dirty colon is that it is an excellent breeding ground for parasites, worms and unfriendly bacteria. When the colon is a cesspool of these organisms, they steal our valuable nutrients and live off them. Some worms get lodged into the fecal mucoid matter so deeply that even strong herbs won't kill them. Some people have done cleanses and found worms from one to 20 feet long. Yuck!

Disease almost always originates in the colon, because when it is overloaded with toxins on a regular basis, those toxins seep into the bloodstream and lymph, eventually settling into weaker areas of the body. The body deliberately stores toxins in fat cells for safekeeping, but when too much builds up in one area, cancer or other serious diseases can develop. The name of the disease depends upon where the poisons settle. In women, one of the largest areas of fat is found in breast tissue—this is why breast cancer is so prevalent. If you understand this one concept—*that most disease originates from a dirty colon (and wrong diet)*—you'll understand more about the cause of degenerative disease than most of the western medical community (which advocates drugs to manage such symptoms, and surgery to cut out affected parts).

When I did my first colon cleanse in 1996, I followed a program based on the suggestions of Dr. Richard Anderson (which I'll share in a moment) for three days, and all kinds of interesting things came out. I knew the program was working when I expelled very foul smelling stuff, because that is the deeply lodged matter in the intestines that normally just sits there and rots. I was surprised, but at the same time delighted, because I knew I was ridding my body of toxins and parasites that weren't doing me any good. After the three days of cleansing, I felt lighter, more energetic, peaceful and centered. The most amazing thing was that I had no idea how "heavy with energy" I was until after the cleanse. Getting rid of that poison was awesome! I now "colon cleanse" on a regular basis.

Cleansing your colon isn't that difficult, but it does require some effort. I'll give a quick overview of the basic concepts here, which you can follow and benefit from. As I mentioned, I strongly suggest reading the book *Cleanse & Purify Thyself* by Dr. Anderson, and acquiring his *Arise & Shine* program (which includes all the ingredients you'll need). I've modified my program from his, but his is an excellent one to start with.

First I'm going to describe the various components of the cleanse, then I'll give you a program you can use.

Hydrated Bentonite Clay

Hydrated bentonite is a clay that comes from volcanic ash. It is often used as a thickener in facial masks because it absorbs excess oil and dirt from the skin. Internal use of volcanic ash goes back to the indigenous peoples of the high Andes Mountains, tribes in Central Africa, and the Aborigines of Australia. When taken internally, it acts like a sponge to bind and eliminate non-nutritive and harmful substances from the colon. It can absorb 180 times or more its own weight of these toxins. Hydrated bentonite is made by suspending microfine, USP-grade bentonite clay in purified water. Bentonite is usually taken with psyllium husk powder.

Mix two tablespoons of the clay with four ounces of water and four ounces of fresh apple juice. Within five minutes of drinking the bentonite "shake," drink a psyllium shake (below).

Psyllium Husk Powder

Psyllium husk powder swells 40 to 60 times its weight when liquid is added. The psyllium binds to the fecal matter as it moves through the intestinal tract—swelling as it absorbs water and waste material in the bowels. This forms a soft, bulky mass that passes through the colon more quickly (keeping potentially toxic waste from staying in the colon) and evacuates more smoothly and easily. The bentonite clay and the psyllium work together synergistically to quickly and efficiently pull out the toxins and the mucoid matter. Psyllium is not digested in the small intestine, but is partially broken down in the colon, where it acts as a food source for friendly flora.

The best way to take psyllium husk powder is to mix two rounded teaspoons with six ounces of warm soy milk—then drink it fast, as it coagulates quickly!

Herbal Cleansers

Prior to and during a colon cleanse, it is wise to take herbs that break up the fecal matter. The herbs prepare the way for the bentonite and psyllium, ensuring that the mucoid matter is more easily dislodged from the intestinal walls. Various natural product manufacturers sell herbal for-

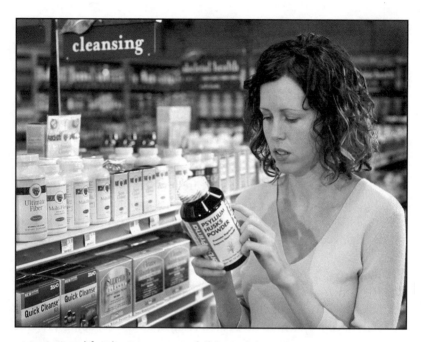

Natural food stores carry a full line of detoxification products.

mulas specifically designed for cleansing. *Arise & Shine*'s product is called "Chomper." *Nature's Secret* has a blend called "Super Cleanse For Your Colon." Some of the herbs commonly used in these formulas are: cascara sagrada bark, fennel seed, ginger root, licorice root, plantain, barberry bark, myrrh, golden seal, capscium, red raspberry leaf and lobelia. It's beyond the scope of this book to describe the benefits of all of these herbs; however, most herbal formulas for colon cleansing will contain the herbs required to break up the fecal mucoid matter and prepare the intestines for the bentonite clay and psyllium husk formula. For the best results, you don't want to skip this step. (Cascara sagrada is a cathartic laxative; it is the active ingredient in Exlax. Cathartic laxatives should be used with caution, as dependency can develop.)

Minerals & Nutritional Support
During a colon cleanse, you should abstain from solid foods. It is very helpful to take supplements that are nutrient-dense, because bentonite

clay not only removes toxins, but also removes minerals that you'll need to replace. I suggest taking one or two green superfoods such as Klamath Lake algae, chlorella or spirulina (I give a full description of these wonder foods in the Supplements section). You can also take a liquid mineral formula. *Arise & Shine* makes one that you can order from their Web site, and several varieties are sold in natural foods stores.

Although you won't be eating solid foods, you can drink freshly pressed vegetable and wheat grass juices. Freshly pressed, organic vegetable juices are packed with vitamins and minerals, help cleanse the intestinal tract and can allay hunger, while fresh wheat grass juice is a natural blood purifier and has an excellent nutritional profile. My favorite juice is a combination of organic carrot, beet, parsley and apple, with a small touch of ginger.

PH Balance

Dr. Richard Anderson suggests you measure the pH (an indicator of acid/alkaline balance) of your saliva to ensure you have enough alkaline minerals in your system to do a colon cleanse; otherwise, doing a cleanse could cause some problems. You can find pH paper at most natural food stores. Don't eat anything for two hours, then wet a strip of the paper with saliva and hold it next to the accompanying color chart. If the reading is between 6.4 and 7.0, you probably have adequate alkaline minerals to do a cleanse. If it's below 6.3, you may want to take the above listed supplements for a week, then take the test again.

Enema and/or Colonic

Flushing out the intestinal tract with water is very highly recommended, because this helps move the fecal matter out faster and more thoroughly. Most people cringe at the idea of doing an enema themselves, or at the thought of a colonic, administered by a colon hydrotherapist, but it's an amazing way to rid the body of unwanted and decaying waste that has been building up in the intestines for years, or even decades. It's a perfect complement to the herbal formulas, bentonite clay and psyllium powder.

While doing a cleanse, flushing out the intestines once a day is advised. Enemas aren't really that difficult, but they do take some time getting used to. And once you experience one, you'll be happy with the results.

You can buy an enema bag at many drugstores. Use cool to room temperature filtered water, if possible, but tap water will do if you don't have a choice. Fill the bag with water and hang it a few feet above ground level. Lubricate the tip of the anal wand with olive oil. You can lie on your back with legs up, or on your side, pulling the top leg close to you for better flow. Insert the tip, and then gently open the valve to allow the water to flow in.

If you've never done this before, it'll feel different, that's for sure. Let the water flow in slowly, but with some pressure. Once it starts feeling uncomfortable, stop the water. Move around a bit to see if the water inside the intestines will flow around blockages, easing the pressure. If the pressure doesn't ease after a moment, or if you feel like you have to "go," then do so. Repeat this process several times until you can get an entire bag of water into your intestines (this is true for most people, but use your own good judgment!) and then release.

You'll want to check out what comes out of you. It's different when you're doing a colon cleanse than when you're eating regular food. And if it's more foul smelling than usual, you know the cleanse is working and that that putrid stuff is finally out of your body!

Not everyone should do an enema. Check first with your primary care provider to determine if this is the best course of action for you.

Three Day Cleanse

During the cleanse you might feel somewhat "spacey" and ungrounded, so I suggest doing it when you have few responsibilities. This is a time of healing, relaxation and reflection. By the way, I would call this an accelerated cleanse, because for aeons spiritual adepts have fasted on water for days or weeks to purify their bodies in order to gain greater attunement to higher vibrations. The cleanse I present is a type of fast, but it includes components which speed up the elimination of undesirable elements lodged in our bodies that can't be achieved by fasting on water alone.

There are many ways to do a cleanse. This basic schedule will get you started; as you learn more you can vary it according to your needs. I suggest you begin with seven days of preparation, followed by three days of the actual cleanse (which is when you are taking only juice, herbs, bentonite clay and psyllium husk powder, and doing the optional enema or colonic).

For the first seven days, eat only organic and plant-based foods as much as possible. Drink some fresh carrot/apple/beet juice, along with two ounces of wheat grass juice every day. Take a daily herbal supplement for colon cleansing, as well as the supplements recommended in this book (see the Supplements chapter).

Three days before the main cleanse, replace one of your meals (probably dinner) with the bentonite and psyllium drinks (taken five minutes apart). Do the same thing two days before the cleanse. One day before the cleanse, replace two meals with the bentonite clay and psyllium husk drinks (again, taken five minutes apart).

For three days, follow this schedule (more or less):

9:00 AM Take herbal & nutritional supplements
11:00 AM Take bentonite clay / psyllium husk powder drinks
1:00 PM Take herbal & nutritional supplements
3:00 PM Take bentonite clay / psyllium husk powder drinks
5:00 PM Take herbal & nutritional supplements
7:00 PM Take bentonite clay / psyllium husk powder drinks
9:00 PM Do an enema (unless visiting a colon hydrotherapist)

You can modify this schedule to two instead of three times a day if that seems more appropriate. It's always best to listen to your body. Remember, this is only a guide—adjust based on how you feel.

If you find you can't think clearly, brown miso broth can be very grounding. You can make your own broth from fermented "pastes." (My favorite brand of miso paste is "Miso Master," found in the refrigerator section at natural foods stores.) If you feel you must eat, try some cooked brown rice, which is also very grounding and has cleansing properties.

The day after the three-day cleanse, begin by eating a small amount of raw plant food, such as a salad. Chew thoroughly. After fasting for three days, you'll find that food tastes more vibrant and flavorful. You'll also find you won't feel like eating as much as you did before.

It's important to take the probiotics I recommend in the Supplements section, because these friendly bacteria are needed to re-colonize your colon after a cleanse.

What to Expect

If you follow the cleanse as outlined above, you'll feel much lighter (energetically) and have more energy afterwards. Your digestive system will be able to absorb more nutrients. The "transit time" of food moving through your intestines will shorten. You will have begun the process of removing disease-causing encrustations from your bowels. Your intestines will begin to regain their normal, healthy state.

This is just the beginning. I suggest doing a three-day cleanse every month for three months, and then see if you can do a five-day cleanse. I felt wonderful after a five-day cleanse. I can't stress enough that cleansing your colon is essential if you want vibrant health!

Parasite & Worm Cleanse

The colon cleanse will help eliminate parasites and worms, but probably won't be able to completely rid you of these critters. Systemic parasites and worms are a greater problem than most people think, including medical doctors. And getting rid of them isn't easy. Some symptoms of these organisms include a voracious appetite, weakness, a withered yellow look, bluish or purplish specks in the whites of the eyes, anal itching, abdominal pain, diarrhea, gas, constipation, cravings for sweet or burnt foods, grinding teeth while sleeping, and a host of others. Parasites affect the body's chemistry and therefore should be eliminated so we can function at our best.

Worms and parasites enter our bodies in a variety of ways, but one of the most common is through uncooked or undercooked meats. We may also be exposed through our pets. Lakes, rivers and tap water are other potential sources of parasites.

Some herbs and supplements used to fight parasites and worms include: black walnut, pumpkin seeds, wormwood, cloves, garlic, raw onions, raw rice, colloidal silver, prickly ash bark and thyme, to name a few. Oxygen therapy can be beneficial. As I said, killing off these critters isn't easy—there is a science to getting rid of them. I suggest either visiting a naturopathic doctor or checking out some of the programs you can find on the Web. Search for "parasite cleanse" and you'll get plenty of programs to choose from. A friend has recommended the products at this web site, www.drnatura.com, for parasite cleansing, though I haven't tried their products.

Lymph Cleanse

The lymphatic system is part of our "garbage-disposal," and is also part of our immune system. The lymph system transports nutrients to cells and removes waste from cells. Unlike blood, lymph fluid can dig deep into tissue to remove toxic waste such as acids and catarrh (mucous). Lymph glands then collect the waste material and dump it into the bloodstream for delivery to the colon, kidneys, lungs or skin for elimination. The lymph vessels also carry special white blood cells (lymphocytes) that challenge and destroy dangerous material before damage can occur.

Unfortunately, this valuable detoxification, nutrient transport and immune building system is often severely neglected. When not properly cared for, the lymph system can be overloaded with toxins, and then health is compromised. However, there is a very simple treatment you can do to help your lymphatic system function properly: exercise.

Daily exercise, especially bouncing on a mini-trampoline (sometimes referred to as a rebounder), will stimulate the lymph fluid and help eliminate harmful toxins from the body. In fact, without exercise, the lymph system barely operates! I suggest 20 minutes of vigorous exercise a day to ensure the lymphatics function correctly.

Apple Cider Vinegar Cleanse

Pure, organic, unfiltered apple cider vinegar has been used successfully for thousands of years to cleanse and purify the body of toxins, facilitating healing. Organic apple cider vinegar has numerous vitamins, minerals and trace minerals, especially potassium, which aids in the cleansing and healing process. Numerous books have been written about the wonders of apple cider vinegar. Drinking a few teaspoons a day will be of great benefit. Just be sure to get pure, organic and unfiltered apple cider vinegar (found in the natural foods section at supermarkets or at natural foods stores) because the highly processed varieties do not have these health benefits. Read more about the benefits of apple cider vinegar in Chapter 6.

Heavy Metal Detox

Many of us have heavy metal poisoning from mercury (from the amalgam in our teeth and other sources), or from too much copper or lead in our body, etc. Heavy metals can cause numerous health problems, as well as psychological troubles. One research study I reviewed said that most violent criminals had elevated levels of heavy metals. One way to learn whether or not you have heavy metal poisoning is to go to a naturopathic doctor (discussed in Chapter 10) and ask for a "hair analysis"—a special test where a laboratory analyzes a small swatch of your hair to reveal the levels of mineral and metal concentrations. Your naturopath may have other tests to run as well to asses your heavy metal levels. Once you have that information, your naturopath will be able to suggest the correct protocol to remove the heavy metal(s) from your system. This is an important part of detoxifying your body, and shouldn't be overlooked.

Skin Cleanse

Sometimes we can neglect the largest organ in the body, our skin, which often exhibits health problems before we sense any symptoms. Keep your skin functioning optimally by using a stiff, natural bristle brush to exfoliate dead cells, allowing your pores to breathe and eliminate properly. Epsom salt baths help draw toxins out of the body, while sea salt and essential oils in the bath water can also be used to pull out toxins. A number of manufacturers sell mixtures of pre-packaged ingredients that you can add to your bath, which can be found in natural food stores.

Conclusion

If you want vibrant health, you simply cannot skip the detox step. I encourage you to try the bentonite clay / psyllium husk cleanse, a colonic or an enema and to drink fresh wheat grass juice (discussed in the Supplements chapter). As I mentioned, I've used Dr. Richard Anderson's *Arise & Shine* system (www.ariseandshine.com) and it worked quite well for me. Dr. Richard Schulze (www.herbdoc.com) also has an excellent and highly effective cleansing program. Natural food stores carry a wide variety of cleansing products as well. I've never had a single person tell me they didn't feel better after doing such cleanse. In fact, they always rave about the positive effects they feel. When you clean out your system, you'll feel better! The detoxification system I've presented has been tested by hundreds of thousands of people. They've had success, and so can you.

8
Exercise
Improve Your Confidence

"You can eat perfectly, but if you don't exercise, you cannot get by.
There are so many health food nuts out there that eat nothing but
natural foods but they don't exercise and they look terrible. Then
there are other people who exercise like a son-of-a-gun but eat a
lot of junk. They look pretty good because exercise is king.
Nutrition is queen. Put them together and you've got a kingdom!"[1]
—Jack LaLanne

Jack said it best, and most of us know that exercising regularly is beneficial to our health. Unfortunately, most of us don't exercise regularly, due to busy schedules or other activities we think have higher priority. Record numbers of Americans are now dangerously obese, due to a combination of poor diet and lack of exercise. I can relate: for most of my life, even after eating a more healthful diet, I avoided regular exercise. Only in the last few years have I begun a consistent program. Since I've been exercising regularly, I find I have better posture and better muscle tone. I feel more confident. Had I known 15 years ago what I *feel* now about the benefits of exercise, I would have motivated myself to begin then.

And motivation is the key. Exercising on a regular basis requires focused thought and determination; it requires an extra expenditure of energy and the effort of creating a new habit. I'll tell you a secret about exercise, though: once you get into a rhythm of doing it at least four or five days a week, and you put out enough effort to work up a sweat for at least 20 to 30 minutes, it gets easier and easier. Not only that, but after you're finished and take that hot shower, you'll feel energized and willing to take on the world. Throughout the day you'll feel stronger and more confident, and the next day, when it's time to exercise again, you'll look forward to it, because you'll know how much better you'll feel (and look!).

There are three keys to exercising effectively:

- Choose an exercise program you enjoy (or you won't stick to it)
- Exercise regularly, preferably three to five times a week
- Do it enough to work up a perspiration for 20 to 30 minutes

You have plenty of options to choose from when it comes to exercise. As I said, it's important to do something you enjoy, and to do it long enough to work up a sweat. Do any of the following appeal to you?

- Sports (basketball, volleyball, tennis, bicycling, in-line skating, etc.)
- Swimming
- Weight / cardiovascular training at a gym
- Martial arts (kung fu, karate, tae kwon do, aikido, among others)
- Specialized resistance training (Pilates, gyrotonics)

All of the above will develop muscle tone, move toxins out of your body and help you feel grounded. Once you've chosen a discipline, stick with it for at least a month; you can always try something else if it isn't working. Of course, if you have particular health concerns or you're pregnant, check with your doctor before beginning an exercise program.

In this chapter I'll give you an overview of the benefits of various types of exercise, including one you may not be familiar with: gyrotonics. I guarantee that once you begin exercising on a regular basis, you'll feel the same exhilaration that I enjoy, along with increased energy and a trimmer waistline!

Health Benefits of Exercise

Regular physical exercise can lower your resting heart rate, which means your heart pumps more blood per beat and is not overworking when you are at rest. Exercise can also lower or help control your blood pressure and reduce your total cholesterol, lowering LDL (the bad type), and increasing HDL (the good type). It also reduces the amount of free fatty acids (triglycerides) in your blood and improves the functioning of your immune system. Exercise reduces the risk of heart disease and stroke, and increases insulin sensitivity to prevent against type II (adult onset) diabetes. The mental and emotional benefits are just as powerful. You can look forward to less anxiety and depression, better stress management and improved self-esteem, appearance, and sleep! Additionally, regular exercise gives you the experience of goal setting and the dedication necessary to achieve your goals—skills you can use in other areas of life. It can be a great help if you're trying to quit smoking or rid yourself of other addictions.

Aerobic Exercise

Let's look at aerobic activities (aerobic means "in the presence of oxygen") first, since this is what most of us need to incorporate into our routine right away. Technically, aerobic exercise improves your body's ability to maximally uptake and deliver oxygen to your working muscles (defined as your "VO2 max"). This is generally regarded as the best measure of your physical fitness level. Aerobic activities elevate your heart rate and breathing for a sustained period, at varying degrees of intensity. It improves the efficiency of your heart and lungs, helps you lose fat and control your weight, and increases muscle and joint flexibility.

Aerobic activities include things like basketball, bicycling, brisk walking, calisthenics, cross-country skiing, dancing, downhill skiing, hiking uphill, jogging, jumping rope, racquetball, roller skating, rowing, running, singles tennis, squash, stair climbing, stationary cycling, step exercise classes, swimming, volleyball, and walking.

If you've been a couch potato (or ill, or inactive for other reasons) for more than a year, you may want to begin with walking. Even five minutes of brisk walking will get you moving in the right direction. Try taking the stairs instead of the elevator at work, or park your car a little further away from the office to get in some "automatic" walking time. Or walk around the block in your neighborhood before or after dinner. The next day, increase it by five minutes or by another block.

If you live in a warm climate, why not choose an activity that will get you outdoors? Join a baseball, basketball or volleyball team that meets at least three times a week. Or take a beach walk/jog one day, go in-line skating another, and swim a third. To be sure you make time for exercise, schedule an appointment for yourself and treat it as you would any other commitment on your calendar. Soon, you'll find it's hard *not* to get out and move.

Choosing A Gym

For those who don't live in year-round outdoor climates, a good gym can be indispensable. Some clubs are even open 24 hours a day, giving you great time flexibility. While joining a gym is an added cost, remember that you are investing in yourself. Look for a "new members special," or ask to have the introductory fee waived (it never hurts to ask, and most gyms will bend over backwards to accommodate your needs). Once you join, you'll find that today's aerobic equipment has come a long way from traditional treadmills and stair-steppers. New, sophisticated machines like elliptical and arc trainers, recumbent bikes and rowing machines (and even the treadmills and stair-steppers have been upgraded) include digital tracking that monitors your heart rate, distance, effort and mileage. They'll tell you when you're on target for fat burning or for cardio training.

Don't be intimidated by buff bodies around you—they're focused on their goals, just like you'll be focused on yours (though you'll probably see all kinds of people in the gym: young, older, fit, fat, disabled, rehabilitating, pregnant, you name it, they're there). Do ask for a knowledgeable gym employee to show you the equipment layout and how to use the machines. And consider investing in a couple of sessions with a personal trainer who can set you up with a personalized routine to meet your goals.

Most gyms offer a variety of aerobics classes tailored for various fitness levels. Read the class descriptions and choose one that meets your needs. Most gyms now offer yoga and Pilates classes as well as kickboxing or *bosu* (short for "both sides up") ball classes, which challenge balance and coordination while giving you a good sweat!

Benefits of Aerobic Exercise:
- Increased maximal oxygen consumption (VO2max)
- Improvement in cardiovascular/cardiorespiratory function (heart and lungs)
- Increased maximal cardiac output (amount of blood pumped every minute)
- Increased maximal stroke volume (amount of blood pumped with each beat)
- Increased blood volume and ability to carry oxygen
- Reduced workload on the heart (myocardial oxygen consumption) for any particular sub-maximal (less than maximum exertion) exercise intensity
- Increased blood supply to muscles and ability to use oxygen
- Lower heart rate and blood pressure at any level of sub-maximal exercise
- Increased threshold for lactic acid accumulation
- Lower resting systolic and diastolic blood pressure in people with high blood pressure
- Increased HDL Cholesterol (the good cholesterol)
- Decreased blood triglycerides
- Reduced body fat and improved weight control
- Improved glucose tolerance and reduced insulin resistance

Anaerobic Exercise (Resistance Training)
There is more to exercise than cardiovascular fitness. Muscle strength is an equally important component to overall personal health and fitness. Anaerobic activities are short in duration, and emphasize building muscle rather than burning oxygen. Anaerobic activities include football, push-ups, sit-ups, soccer, softball, sprinting and weight lifting. Strength training is anything that causes resistance against body movements in order to strengthen muscles. Examples are workouts with barbells, dumbbells, Universal gyms or Nautilus equipment.

Strength training provides three primary benefits:
1. Enhancement/Maintenance of Lean Muscle Weight
Everyone loses a half-pound of muscle every year after age 20 unless they incorporate some strength training into their exercise routine.

2. Injury Prevention and Increased Capacity
Strengthening major muscle groups lessens impact stresses and the risk of
exercise-related injury. Strong muscles also help you do daily tasks with
ease and efficiency. Climbing stairs, lifting groceries, cleaning the house,
and mowing the lawn all become easier.

3. Prevention of Osteoporosis
Most anaerobic activities are load-bearing exercises that promote bone
growth.

Additional benefits of strength training:
- Increased muscular strength
- Increased strength of tendons and ligaments
- Improved range of motion of joints
- Reduced body fat and increased lean body mass (muscle mass)
- Can decrease resting systolic and diastolic blood pressure
- Positive changes in blood cholesterol
- Improved glucose tolerance and insulin sensitivity
- Improved strength, balance, and functional ability in older adults

Endorphins—Your Body's Natural High
The increase in endorphins generated when you exercise is a great reward
for your effort. It's the "runner's high" we've all heard about. But what
exactly are endorphins, and what is their role in the human body? In
1972, Dr. Candace Pert discovered the "opiate receptor" within the human brain. This meant that the brain must secrete a morphine-like substance (appropriately named "endorphin" for "morphine within") since it
has such receptors. When activated, these receptors block pain signals to
the nervous system, providing the body with a natural pain reliever that
also causes a euphoric effect.

Twenty different types of endorphins (also known as "enkephalins")
have been discovered in the nervous system. One, beta-endorphin, is
18 to 50 times more effective than morphine, while another, called di-
morphic, is over 500 times stronger. Endorphins, however, are unable to
work for long periods of time because our bodies also make endorphins
enzymes, which eradicate them (another reason for daily exercise).

Endorphins may act as more than just a built-in-pain-control system. Some scientists claim that endorphins enhance our immune system and block the lesion of blood vessels, thereby lowering blood pressure. Furthermore, by also removing super-oxides (molecules that attack living tissue, causing disease and aging), endorphins have anti-aging effects.

Pilates and Gyrotonics

I want to introduce you to two specialized forms of fitness training: "Pilates" and "gyrotonics." Developed nearly 100 years apart, both methods are now becoming popular and offer the exceptional benefits once reserved for professionals or the elite among us.

Pilates

The Pilates method is a unique system of stretching and strengthening exercises. It was developed over 90 years ago by Joseph Pilates, who was born in Germany in the 1880s and suffered from asthma, rickets and rheumatic fever as a child. He began exercising and bodybuilding to overcome his physical limitations, and in his early teens became a model for anatomical drawings and enjoyed many sports, including gymnastics. At age 32, he moved to England and worked as a self-defense instructor at Scotland Yard. He was interned as an enemy alien at the outbreak of World War I, during which time he refined his ideas and, using springs on hospital beds, developed exercise equipment to help rehabilitate wounded soldiers. After the war, he moved to the U.S. and opened an exercise studio in New York. His technique became popular with dancers and was adopted in dance training regimens around the world.

For many years, Pilates training remained a well-kept secret among dancers and other performing artists. The growing interest in mind/body exercise has brought Pilates concepts to the forefront of fitness training. This method encompasses more than 500 exercises (don't worry, you don't do them all every time), performed as a mat-based workout or using special resistance equipment. Pilates stretches and tones muscles while reducing tension and strain in the joints and lower back.

Gyrotonics

This unique exercise system has been described as "yoga with resistance." Juliu Horvath, a principal dancer in the world renowned Rumanian State Opera, developed gyrotonics ("gyro"—ring, spiral or circle, and "tonic"—to tone or invigorate), based on yoga, ballet, swimming, dance, tai chi and gymnastics in the late 1980s at the White Cloud Studio in NYC.

The fluid sequence of exercises is performed on a Horvath designed apparatus—the gyrotonics tower/handle machine—that uses hand-and foot-operated wheelbases and suspended pulleys to create resistance. There are 50 sets of exercises (with approximately 130 variations) to stretch, bend, twist and turn muscles with minimal effort. Unlike most conventional exercise machines that encourage linear or isolated movement patterns, gyrotonic exercises encourage a complete range of circular motion and full articulation of stabilized joints. All major muscle groups are worked interdependently and are synchronized with a corresponding breathing pattern. They are performed rhythmically, creating gentle or vigorous cardiovascular-aerobic stimulation, depending on intensity and speed. Special attention is placed on increasing the functional capacity of the spine, resulting in a well-proportioned body that is significantly less prone to injuries.

Conclusion

As I said earlier, I wish I had begun exercising 15 years ago. Nevertheless, I exercise now and am thankful that I'm finally doing it on a regular basis. So, don't feel bad about yourself if you haven't started yet; rather, make the commitment to do the research and find the right exercise for you, and then begin. Better late than never is always the case, and I assure you that you'll live your life with more energy and confidence after you've adopted a regular exercise program.

9
Chi Energy
Build Your Personal Power

While exercise has a measurable effect on our physiology and improves our physical, mental and emotional health, there is another component necessary for true fitness. It's known as "vital life force," "qi," "chi," "prana," "divine essence"— and it's what animates all living things. Though it's invisible, it's something we feel every day. Can't wait to do something? Your chi is probably strong. Can't get out of bed? It's probably weak. Angry, frustrated or depressed? It's probably stuck. Our attitudes, emotions and sense of well-being are all influenced by our chi. In Oriental medicine, strong chi is synonymous with excellent health, mental clarity and physical vitality. A weakened or blocked flow of this vital essence is considered the beginning of all disease. Acupuncture is effective because it acts at this "energetic" level. When you cultivate and build your chi, you build your personal power.

While it's thought that we're born with a limited amount of genetic chi, we can cultivate "acquired" chi through our lifestyle choices. The idea is to balance active and receptive energies, which we can do by getting enough rest, eating well and balancing exercise and recreational activities with those that specifically enhance chi reserves and flow. Interestingly, this vital energy isn't necessarily enhanced by exercise. Over-exercise or exercising with poor posture or muscular imbalances can actually weaken your life force.

In this chapter I discuss this animating principle in more detail, then look at five different disciplines that can add the "chi factor" to your life. Yoga, an ancient practice enjoying Western popularity, offers seemingly unlimited styles for any shape, size or personality type. Qigong, "the grandfather of martial arts," can build strength from the inside out, while tai chi chuan (tai chi), known as "moving meditation," is a gentle introduction to the martial arts, and a great way to build and balance chi. Aikido, "the way of harmonizing with the infinite," shows that self-defense can be gentle and graceful as well as efficacious. Kung Fu, the most intense way to build chi, appeals to the athletically inclined and will challenge you at every level. Any of these arts will complement your exercise program to uplift your body, mind and spirit and nourish your chi.

Extraordinary Chi

The ability to focus and guide chi can lead to extraordinary power and an extremely high pain threshold. A parent lifting a car off a child in an emergency is an example of strong chi (and, of course an adrenaline rush!) in action. The "flying technique" portrayed in the film *Crouching Tiger, Hidden Dragon* is an example of an extreme focus of such energy. This "chi power" is perhaps most dramatically illustrated by the strength of older, frail-looking martial arts masters calmly fending off two or more larger, younger opponents with barely the blink of an eye. Sometimes the force emitted from such a master is strong enough to physically knock the opponent down before he even reaches the master.

Yoga

Yoga is offered in most gyms these days, and yoga studios are popping up everywhere, even in rural communities. There are many styles (Astanga, Bikram, Iyengar, Kripalu, Yin Yoga and Viniyoga to name just a few), but all of them are forms of Hatha Yoga. This wonderful self-care system originated in India; the names of the postures are in Sanskrit, an ancient Indian language. "Ha" means sun; "tha" means moon. Together they express a wholeness of polarities, like the Oriental yin/yang balance. (See Chapter 5 for a more thorough discussion of the principles of yin and yang.)

Yoga postures can be used to strengthen and stretch muscles, joints and connective tissue. The emphasis on lengthening the spine in every pose—combined with twisting postures—irrigates vertebrae, keeping them youthful even into old age. The poses, (called "asanas") promote the flow of energy through the nervous system and assist in the elimination of toxins. They exert a beneficial pressure on glands and internal organs, flushing and stimulating them.

Yoga prevents, relieves or eliminates many symptoms and conditions, including hypertension, arthritis, osteoporosis and diabetes. The discipline also affords mental and emotional fitness. Most people experience a deep sense of well being after the first class, departing with a sense of relaxation and clarity of mind. Others experience emotional "cleansing," as deeply repressed feelings are released to the surface. On a psychological level, yoga can be a profound tool, gently uncovering negative patterns and offering more comfortable, spacious ways of being with yourself and others.

For those on a spiritual path, the discipline of a regular yoga practice provides a foundation for the trek. The word yoga means "union." For some, that means union with the divine; for others, it may be uniting hands to feet. But beyond stretching, beyond strengthening, yoga clears pathways within the body. Your natural chi energy can then flow straight through you, like a laser beam of light, illuminating the way.

The multi-dimensional benefits of yoga have been recognized in Germany, Australia and England for use in medical treatment protocols. Here in the United States, Dr. Dean Ornish has established a rehabilitative program for cardiac patients which includes yoga and meditation as pivotal factors in reversing heart disease.

Developing Chi Through Martial Arts
One of the best ways to develop chi is by practicing a martial art. There are literally hundreds to choose from; in fact, more than 300 different styles are practiced in China, where most of them originated. Interestingly, Chinese martial arts arose from the same roots as Chinese medicine. Martial artists were trained in medicine, while doctors were trained in martial arts. Priests and monks were both doctors and martial artists, and were practitioners of "energy medicine."

Chinese martial arts are differentiated as being either external or internal. Named for their area of origin, the external arts use muscular force, speed and sheer strength to produce power. They emphasize linear movements, high impact contact, jumps, and kicks. Internal martial arts use what the Chinese call "wise force" to overcome opponents. They combine internal chi energy with muscle strength to produce power. Tai chi, Aikido and Kung Fu are internal arts. Along with fighting techniques, internal training often includes standing meditation and exercises to develop chi.

Qigong

Qigong can be considered the root, or "grandfather" of not only all forms of martial arts, but also of Chinese healing systems. This ancient practice of healing, health maintenance and self-development dates back thousands of years; it involves posture, movement, self-massage, breathing techniques, and meditation. The specific practices are designed to cultivate, increase, and refine chi. Impure or stale energy is eliminated, while the flow of healthy, pure chi is enhanced. You don't need a large space or special equipment, and it's easy to learn.

The ultimate goal is to fully develop your body, mind and spirit. With training and experience, you can use qigong for self-healing. When it's used to heal others, the practice is known as medical qigong. There may be thousands of different "schools," and the many styles are based on some common principles and practices. Qigong teachers often come from a long lineage of a particular style.[1]

Tai Chi Chuan (Tai Chi)

If you're looking for a non-impact workout, tai chi chuan (known also as tai chi) may be the perfect choice. Some say it's the oldest of the martial arts; it's been practiced in China for centuries and is popular in both rural and industrial areas there today. Originally, tai chi was a fighting form that emphasized strength, balance, flexibility, and speed. Adversarial energy was redirected back to the sender so that an opponent could experience his or her own negative intentions. Today, this art is almost exclusively practiced as therapeutic exercise and meditation, characterized by slow, gentle movements.

Based on the principle of yin and yang, in which opposing but complementary forces combine to create harmony, tai chi developed into a movement and breathing system that exercised all the joints and major muscle groups while circulating internal energy. It is this circulation of chi that prevents or mitigates disease and promotes health. Tai chi increases strength, stamina, and flexibility, and is easy on joints. It cultivates the link between mind and body, enhancing balance and coordination. It also reduces blood pressure, improves oxygen utilization and immune function, increases bone density, and reduces stress hormone levels. Many of these effects have been documented in elderly beginners practicing an abbreviated form for only a few months. If tai chi can have this effect on geriatric beginners, think of what it can do for someone who starts decades sooner!

As with other martial arts, there are many styles and forms. Fundamental to all forms, however, is finding our center, called the "tan tien," or "reservoir." We tap into this source of energy deep inside and practice moving it throughout our bodies to heal and nourish the internal organs, and to balance the immune and endocrine systems. When we consciously direct our movements, we can consciously direct our energy. Some people become so adept at this that they can consciously move chi through the subtle channels known as acupuncture meridians.

Tai chi emphasizes continuous, flowing movement. There's no over-extension or wasted effort—the whole body moves in unison, each part balanced by another-gently rotating and transforming into the next movement. Unlike other forms of exercise, Tai chi doesn't cause panting or breathlessness; breathing deepens as tension is released.

Aikido

Aikido is a relatively new self-defense art. It was founded in Japan by Professor Morihei Ueshiba (1883-1969). As a youth, Ueshiba spent years of intense training in budo, a Japanese martial arts. He was a master of Jiu-jitsu, and was considered unbeatable. As he learned some of the most sophisticated and devastating fighting techniques of Japan, he questioned their intense aggression and the need to defeat others. Inspired by Zen Buddhism and Shinto, an ancient Japanese religion based on love and harmony with nature, Ueshiba sought a more peaceful martial art. He realized that true self-defense was not winning over others, but winning over the discord within oneself. He developed *Aikido*, which means "the way of harmonizing with the spirit of the universe." The study of Aikido involves positive character-building ideals along with self-defense techniques.

Although many Aikido moves resemble the techniques and throws of Jiu Jutsu and Judo, this art focuses on controlling the vital energy centered in the abdominal region in order to subdue an opponent. While Judo's main techniques are throwing, grappling, and attacking vital points, Aikido techniques deflect blows and check offensive attacks by meeting rather than blocking blows. Aikido emphasizes nerve points that, when pressed, can bring down an adversary without risk of maiming or killing. The focus is on freeing yourself from grips, throwing an opponent to the ground by exerting precise leverage maneuvers, then immobilizing the adversary by placing pressure on the joints. Students practice forms by alternatively taking the roles of attacker and defender. There is no competition in Aikido; however, ranks are attained in a process similar to judo, and are awarded at formal demonstrations. Some forms include a long staff (called a bo) or a rubber knife.

During practice, students match their movements to those of others, avoiding collisions and conflicts. They discover their own strengths and weaknesses, mastering themselves as they master the art. Aikido is more than a system of self-defense; it promotes peace and harmony among people. It is a spiritual as well as a physical discipline, and is extremely popular around the world, since it does not require great physical strength and can be practiced effectively by women and the elderly.

Kung Fu

Kung Fu (Chinese boxing) shares, along with Karate, the distinction of being one of the two most popular martial arts. It employs kicks, crouches, strikes, throws, body turns, dodges, holds, leaps and falls, handsprings and somersaults. This style of martial arts (especially Shaolin Kung Fu) is one of the fiercest and most revered. "Black belts" can harness the focus and control to break a solid brick with a bare hand.

Whereas Karate moves are deliberate, forceful and distinct (punches are linear, kicks are in a straight line, and the body is held rigidly), Kung Fu is smooth and fluid—movements meld imperceptibly into one long, graceful action. Properly coordinated chi creates the fluidity associated with Kung Fu. This martial art requires a strict code of physical and mental discipline unparalleled in Western sports. Kung Fu priests of ancient times were adept in art, medicine, music, religions, animal husbandry, cartography, languages, history, the making of weapons and fighting techniques. The artist had to be more than a fighting machine—he had to know how, where and when to enter a fight, and more importantly, how to avoid conflict. Ironically, only with unbeatable ability was he secure enough *not* to need to fight.

The self mastery gained from the study and practice of Kung Fu can become an asset you can use in personal, professional, academic and social situations. The skills learned become part of you, a way of being in the world.

Build Your Personal Power

Though it takes patience and perseverance, cultivating chi energy will be an investment you'll reap rewards from for the rest of your life. It is, after all, what animates all living things. From a single-celled amoeba to the farthest galaxy, chi is behind the scenes creating all the action. Enjoy your exploration of this mysterious, yet tangible force, and build your own personal power.

10
Medicine
Help Your Body Heal Itself

When we are ill, a number of treatment options are available to us. The purpose of this section is to help you understand the differences between the two primary medical philosophies being practiced in the United States today: allopathic (conventional) medicine, and preventive/holistic medicine (also known as natural medicine, or complementary and alternative medicine (CAM)). The conventional Western allopathic system focuses on *disease management*, whereas the older, more established natural system focuses on treating the root cause(s) of disease in order to reestablish health.

This chapter contains an in-depth explanation of several branches of holistic medicine, including acupuncture, Ayurveda, naturopathy, homeopathy, chiropractic, network spinal analysis and massage. I also discuss the facts about the ways in which various branches and practitioners of holistic medicine have been suppressed and harassed by the conventional medical establishment and our government, and then ignored by the media. This persecution helps to keep the mainstream public ignorant and skeptical of the very real benefits that holistic medicine has to offer.

Please keep in mind that the information contained in this chapter concerns the prevention and/or treatment of chronic conditions (heart disease, cancer, hypoglycemia, acne, the flu, etc.), *not* acute injuries (e.g. car accidents, burns, heat exhaustion, frostbite, etc.). Broad generalizations are made throughout this chapter to emphasize points, so please remember that there are always exceptions to my statements. Although I present challenging viewpoints in this chapter, I believe it is in our best interest to wisely use the best of both systems for optimum diagnosis, treatment and healing. And though I'm tough on the modern medical model, implicating its underlying financial motives, I'd like to acknowledge the many dedicated doctors, nurses, technicians and emergency personnel who are true healers working within an established system that is entrenched in a not altogether healthy "feedback loop."

Allopathic Medicine—Symptom/Disease Management

The allopathic medical philosophy taught at most medical schools, and practiced by the majority of medical doctors, relies on the concept of identifying diseases or symptoms, and then prescribing drugs to manage or combat those conditions. It is a system that considers the disease or symptom to be the *actual problem*, as opposed to addressing the *underlying causes* that produced the disease or symptom in the first place. A wide variety of tests, procedures and equipment specially designed to identify diseases and symptoms have been developed, which on one level is great, because these tests could be used to help figure out underlying causes. Yet, on another level they are very limiting, since they are rarely used for such purposes. Typically, once a diagnosis is determined, the tests are plunked into the patient's file as conclusive evidence of his or her condition.

This model considers bacteria, viruses, fungi, molds and other foreign invaders to be some of the main causes of our illnesses; therefore, antibiotics, and/or drugs are prescribed to fight them. In fact, the standard treatment procedure is often the use of drugs to "manage" or "fight," or in many cases to resort to surgery to cut out the problem. Unfortunately, drugs often harm the body with what we term *side effects*. Words and names are powerful concepts in our consciousness. The language of modern allopathic medicine is filled with images of war: the war on cancer, for example. Verbs like control, combat, fight and irradiate connote strife. Invaders must be conquered.

Yet when it comes to drugs, language is more euphemistic. If we said that the drugs are *poisoning* us rather than giving us *side effects*, we might not be so apt to use them on a long-term basis. For example, look through any mainstream magazine, find an ad for a popular drug, and then flip the page to read the extensive list of *side effects*—that's what happens when the body is poisoned over time with drugs.

Since the allopathic medical *model* (notice I said "model," and not "doctor") isn't concerned with getting to the root causes of symptoms and diseases (e.g. the cause of the symptom), it is a *highly profitable* venture due to *repeat clients*. The long-term use of drugs ensures that people never quite get better, and slowly deteriorate due to poor immune function and the side effects of the drugs. As time goes by, more problems are "discovered," so more drugs are prescribed. At some point the conditions can become so severe that the only option available is surgery, which provides more financial windfall. This well-tuned, multi-billion dollar industry is comprised of medical doctors, technicians, hospitals, pharmaceutical empires, government agencies like the FDA, and private organizations such as The American Medical Association, American Dental Association, American Cancer Society, etc. This entire interlocking disease *management* system is designed to provide repeat customers for a very long time—the longer and the more sick we are, the more money to make—a perfect business model!

Medical doctors are *trained to believe* that the system of medicine they are taught is the only valid one (developed by the AMA and its universities), and that natural medicine is more or less just quackery. The Federal Drug Administration (FDA) supports this disease/symptom management industry and works to legally banish, suppress, slander or harass those who use successful natural treatments (particularly cancer cures). They imprison doctors who perform them (see the next section), because such treatments and cures undermine the finances of the allopathic medical conglomerate. Prevention is barely in their vocabulary.

To review, the allopathic medical *model* of diagnosing and treating most chronic conditions relies on procedures and techniques that usually don't address the core issues of why the disease or symptom appeared in the first place. It uses synthetic drugs and surgery to conquer and control the situation—this is called disease/symptom management. For *acute* care, where trauma is involved (such as with a car accident), temporary management of bodily systems is helpful and can even be required for the body to be stabilized (although using natural remedies would also be beneficial). However, long-term use of drugs for *chronic* diseases (heart disease, cancer, high blood pressure, asthma, etc.) only manages *symp-*

toms, doesn't address the root cause(s) and usually toxifies the body. The toxic effects of medical drugs kill over 100,000 people a year.[1] Natural therapies are very safe in comparison, are often more effective, and can even help cure the underlying problem.

Natural Medicine Leads to Real Cures

In contrast, the philosophy of natural medicine holds that a weakened immune system (and/or along with other weakened bodily systems) is the reason foreign invaders can thrive, producing symptoms and diseases.

Most of us are taught that we need to go to medical doctors when we get sick. What we aren't taught is that the *real doctor* is already within us as the *innate wisdom of the body*. This is the difference between conventional allopathic systems and natural holistic medicine systems. The philosophy of natural medicine is that, given the *right conditions*, the body will *heal itself*. Whereas the allopathic model tries to control defective body systems through drug intervention, or kill foreign invaders with antibiotics, natural medicine rarely includes toxic agents. Instead, herbs, homeopathic remedies and other non-invasive therapies are used. These techniques harmoniously help facilitate the repair and strengthening of bodily systems (especially the immune system, which can then properly fight foreign invaders), or help to destroy offending pathogens without toxic side effects. The goal of natural medicine is to figure out why systems have weakened and then repair them, which results in healing.

In natural medicine, prevention is always considered the first priority. Therefore, much attention is placed on *educating the patient* about proper diet and other lifestyle choices that affect health, such as discussed in this book. An ounce of prevention is truly worth a pound of cure, and more. Speaking of cures, only the body cures. Not drugs, not diet, not herbs, or anything else. It is the innate wisdom of the body and the unblocked flow of life force energy that moves through the body that produces healing (cure). However, that doesn't mean we can't *help* the body heal, which is the focus of this book.

Since our bodies do have the innate wisdom to heal themselves, the task of the natural doctor is to figure out how, why and where the body's ecology/energy is out of harmony, and then offer ways to bring it back into harmony through non-toxic means. Healing will almost always occur when bodily systems are brought back into harmony with each other and pathogens are dealt with properly (via toxic-free methods). For example, consider an ear infection, which is very common in children. The allopathic model recommends treatment with antibiotics. That's treating the symptom. The infection may go away, but the underlying cause of the infection—a weakened immune system *and the reason behind the weak immune system*—is still there. Furthermore, antibiotics not only kill offending bacteria in the ear, but often kill immune building bacteria in the gut, creating a downward spiral of reoccurring ear infections and antibiotic treatment. This can ultimately lead to the invasive procedure of intubation (which can and often does lead to ADD/ADHD by seriously compromising the vestibular system housed in the inner ear—see www.handle.org for more information).

On the other hand, natural medical philosophy will question why the immune system has dropped to such a degree that an ear infection took hold in the first place. The underlying cause of the weakened immune system could be a milk allergy (or any allergy, for that matter), poor nutrition, or any number of things, which the natural doctor seeks to discover and then correct—strengthening the immune system as she treats the symptoms of the infection. Treatment of the ear infection itself may include the use of non-toxic herbal formulas, such as garlic and mullein (also found at natural food stores), to destroy harmful bacteria. This helps to stop the current ear infection and the other treatment helps to strengthen the immune system so future occurrences of ear infections become very unlikely—in effect, "curing" the infection.

As you can see, natural healing philosophy embraces quite a number of concepts, which is why you find the word holistic used so frequently. This is because the root cause of a symptom or disease is often a *combination of factors* and optimum health is regained when *multiple* treatment protocols are followed. By following the natural living lifestyle as outlined in this book, you are also following natural healing philosophy because they are inter-linked. First and foremost, holistic/natural ideology is about prevention. If disease does occur, then using remedies that work in harmony with nature—and therefore the body—to rebuild and strengthen weak systems (again, particularly the immune system) and organs is wise.

As a business model, this philosophy offers the natural physician modest financial reward, the satisfaction that clients have regained their health and, often, long-term relationships with clients. From the allo-pathic perspective, natural medicine represents an intrusion on their business of making money off perpetually sick people, so there is often suppression of natural medicine through the established allopathic medi-cal profession. Of course, that's not all. When people adopt the natural living lifestyle, they stop eating the majority of products found in con-ventional grocery stores, causing even more business woes for multi-na-tional corporations. Thus, it's in the best interest of big business, hospi-tals, medical doctors, pharmaceutical empires, the media and allopathic medical organizations to suppress, discredit and even outlaw or severely regulate natural medicine as much as possible.

Suppression of Natural Medicine
From 1257 to 1812 the Inquisition in Europe tortured, burned and murdered over nine million women because they were considered to be witches. Their real crime? They were healers—midwives and herbalists—who knew how to work with nature to produce healing. The Church had decided that sickness was an act of God as punishment for sin, and there-fore discouraged the use of medicine. In the 13th century the Church finally accepted medicine, but only when practiced by men, and only by men with a diploma from a university (the word college, synonymous with 'university,' comes from the Latin College of Cardinals, an intrinsic part of the Church's patriarchal hierarchy). The men gained great power, while the populace and predominantly female healers suffered terribly, and only the ruling elite benefited. The persecution of women, and of true healers, has never quite stopped.[2]

During the 19th century, homeopathy (a discipline of natural medi-cine) flourished, and death rates from cholera, typhoid, and scarlet fever in homeopathic hospitals were between 1/2 and 1/8 of those in conven-tional (allopathic) hospitals. Yet, when the American Medical Association was founded in 1847, a clause was placed in its code of ethics stating that any member who consulted with a homeopath would be kicked out of the membership. Doctors who did were indeed banished from the newly formed, powerful organization.

Until 1910, holistic therapies were taught in most medical schools, while the extensive use of drugs as therapy was taught in just a few. That changed when John D. Rockefeller and the AMA hired Abraham Flexner, a high school teacher, to "evaluate" the effectiveness of therapies taught in medical schools around the country. His findings were published in the *Flexner Report*, which basically denounced natural/holistic therapies and embraced drug-based medicine. Congress followed the recommendations of the report and empowered the American Medical Association (AMA) to certify or de-certify any medical school in the country on the grounds of whether or not that school met the AMA's standards of "approved" medicine. Thus, the natural/holistic healing schools and communities were decimated, and the number of medical schools dropped from 600 to 50 within 15 years (by 1925).[3] The AMA gained a new foothold of power to decide what is and isn't medicine, and has worked ever since to discredit, persecute and outlaw natural therapies. In 1977 the *Declaration of Alma Ata* gave the World Health Organization (controlled by the United Nations) the means to extend the *Flexner Report* not only in North America, but throughout the entire world![4]

The Attack on Chiropractic
During the 1950s, sixties and seventies, chiropractic care became increasingly popular and available because of widespread therapeutic success. This raised the ire of the AMA, and in the early sixties they began a vicious attack on chiropractors specifically, and other holistic/natural healers indirectly, with the intent *to shut down the professions entirely*.[5] Agents of the AMA contacted hundreds of medical groups and societies and urged them to deem it unethical for physicians to refer patients to chiropractors. The AMA began printing malicious, unsubstantiated claims about chiropractors in their consumer publications, using words like "fraud," "hoax" and "cult."

In 1976, three chiropractors had had enough of the harassment. They filed a lawsuit against the AMA and 11 other related medical institutions, alleging that they had all taken part, in various ways, in an illegal conspiracy to destroy the chiropractic profession. During the ensuing 10 years plus trial, the AMA and other defendants claimed that chiropractic care was invalid, but time after time their claims were successfully refuted by chiropractic's obvious successes and the science behind those successes. On August 24, 1987, U.S. District Judge Susan Getzendanner ruled that the AMA and its officials were guilty of attempting to eliminate the chiropractic profession. In November, 1990 the U.S. Supreme Court up-

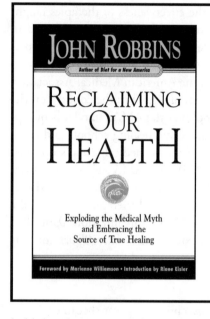

— A MUST READ —

John Robbins exposes the dark side of the allopathic medical establishment's monopoly in his superbly researched book, *Reclaiming Our Health*. He offers insight into the various alternative treatments which the Establishment would prefer remain unknown. Read this excellent book to really understand the forces behind the scenes trying to stop natural medicine.

held that decision, and the AMA agreed to pay 3.5 million dollars for the chiropractors' legal fees and to revise its position.[6]

Midwives Persecuted

Midwives—professionally trained women who help other women give birth naturally (within or outside a hospital environment)—gained popularity during the sixties and seventies. Unfortunately, they were also (and continue to be) attacked by the medical profession on a regular basis (witch-hunts all over again!), which included raids on their homes, arrests and the shutting down of their businesses. For example, when physicians from a local hospital in Santa Cruz, California discovered that midwives were taking business away from them, they organized and declared that midwifery was a public menace. The doctors refused to help in any way with blood tests or other treatments. The midwives found other means to acquire the necessary services, which really infuriated the doctors. [And in 1975, Yale University Hospital told their physicians that they wouldn't be allowed to practice there if they assisted midwives. Other hospitals quickly followed suit.]

The Santa Cruz women faced trumped up charges brought against them by undercover agents sent in at the behest of the physicians. The midwives involved had helped birth more than 300 babies with no deaths and no complaints; yet the local hospital had a mortality rate of three out of 300. At the trial, supporters of the midwives flooded the courtroom. Three years after the arrest (which had used 13 people and eight squad cars to arrest two women on a misdemeanor) the prosecuting attorney dropped the charges. Unfortunately, it took quite a toll on the women involved, financially and emotionally, and they shut down their business. This story is typical throughout the country. Hundreds of midwives all across the nation have been or are still harassed, shut down or thrown in jail for helping other women give birth naturally (pregnancy is considered a disease by the AMA)!

John Robbin's excellent book, *Reclaiming Our Health*, cites numerous examples of present-day midwife persecution, along with sobering evidence of how natural cures for cancer and other diseases are banned by the allopathic medical conglomerate.

Cancer Cures Condemned

Did you know it's illegal to cure cancer? Successful alternative treatments for cancer *really* upsets the FDA, AMA, American Cancer Society, National Cancer Institute, hospital administrators, technicians, pharmaceutical empires and medical doctors. Conventional cancer treatment is a huge industry that stands to lose billions of dollars when holistic cures work. So when people come up with successful cures, they are hounded by the authorities until they are shut down or thrown in jail.

Cancer is not that difficult to understand: it is the result of an overly toxic body, weakened bodily systems and a weakened immune system. Malfunction of the pancreas is believed by some to be one of the leading causes of the development of cancer. Cancer is the result of years or decades of eating polluted food and improper nutrition. When the body can no longer defend itself against the toxins or store them safely in fat cells, the area is overwhelmed and cancer develops. Many holistic physicians believe that cancer is completely reversible through non-toxic treatment. Western allopathic treatments use radiation, chemotherapy (drugs that pull in billions of dollars a year worldwide) and surgery to kill or cut out the pathogens/cancer cells. The result? An immune system seriously compromised or wiped out, as well as other bodily systems severely compromised or wiped out. Next result? Rare recovery or shortened lifespan and probable cancer recurrence, since the *root problem* is not addressed. The payoff? Western medical systems make billions off disease management while patients trapped in the system continue to spiral downward both physically and financially.

The natural approach to cancer is to help the body rebuild its immunity and other bodily systems, so that we can *naturally* overcome the cancerous situation. Most alternative treatments *also* use techniques to kill offending cancer cells and viruses (ozone therapy, herbs, oxygen therapy, etc.) that enhance rather than destroy the immune system. The result? People regain their lives because they learn how to properly care for their health while keeping their immune system intact to prevent a recurrence. The payoff to natural doctors? Knowledge that they are helping people get well. The payoff to the allopathic system of disease management? None.

In the 1950s Harry Hoxsey operated 17 alternative health clinics in 17 states. He was using an herbal formula that thousands of his patients claimed had cured them of cancer. The AMA launched a vicious attack against him and he was subsequently arrested over 100 times! Yet, no cancer patient of his *ever* testified against him, and in fact, every time he was thrown in jail, hundreds of his patients would surround the jail and sing and pray until he was released! Many reporters and other professionals went to him to expose him as a hoax, but wound up vigorously defending him once they learned of his character and treatments.

The attacks on him by the AMA and the police department continued. Finally, he sued the AMA for slander and libel. He became the first person to win a judgement against the AMA. In 1953, Benedict Fitzgerald, Jr., special counsel to the U.S. Senate Commerce Committee, conducted an in-depth investigation and concluded that the FDA, AMA and the National Cancer Institute *conspired* to suppress a fair investigation of Hoxsey's treatments. By 1953 his clinics were flourishing and he had successfully treated over 12,000 people. Unfortunately, in 1960 the FDA found a way to shut down all 17 clinics: they stated that there is no known cure for cancer and therefore that what he was doing was illegal!

Hoxsey's chief nurse moved to Tijuana, Mexico and opened the clinic there, where it continues to thrive and successfully treat people with cancer. Their clinic can be found at: www.cancure.org/hoxsey_clinic.

htm.[7] Cancer treatments that work (and there are many) continue to be suppressed to this day, and people who practice them are persecuted and hounded with a vengeance.

Natural Treatment Suppression and the Media

I could go on and on with stories about how the AMA, FDA and other medical institutions/government agencies deliberately suppress bona fide natural treatments (and you can read dozens of such stories of overt suppression of legitimate treatments in John Robbin's *Reclaiming Our Health*), but the point I want to make is that you probably haven't heard about these methods because the mainstream media is tied to the allopathic medical model. If the allopathic group says it's quackery, then the media will give lip service to the natural treatment, but will always conclude its report in favor of the Establishment, which condemns such therapies with words like *unscientific, anecdotal, false, new-age,* or simply *untrue.* So, you can't look to the mainstream media and expect to hear about truly innovative and effective natural therapies—the same groups of people who own the media also own and intersect with the allopathic medical establishment. And, I must point out that there ARE bogus (so-called) "natural" treatments that don't work, which is why I'm going to give you a quick overview of research based natural medicine remedies and philosophies so you know how to find and use the legitimate ones.

Natural Healing Systems

As I mentioned earlier, holistic doctors use methods and techniques that help the body balance, rebuild and strengthen systems to bring about healing. There are dozens of natural healing models to choose from and, although I respect most of the modalities available, there are a few I believe deserve special mention because of the extensive education involved, as well as the proven success rate.

In my opinion, naturopathic doctors, traditional Chinese medical doctors and acupuncturists are at the top of the list. This is because they have the most education, the widest knowledge base and also have access to diagnostic tests that are not available to other natural practitioners. Next are chiropractors and/or network spinal analysis practitioners (a form of gentle chiropractic), because their type of care helps to ensure the proper nerve signal flow that is so essential to a healthy body. If I had a medical condition, I would seek the counsel of a member of one or more of the "top tier" above; then, as money and time permitted, I would seek additional natural therapies (such as massage, herbal remedies, nutritional counseling, energetic healing, etc.).

Traditional Chinese medicine (TCM) and acupuncture are based on an "energetic" model of healthcare. A practitioner of this discipline is interested in how well energy (called chi or qi) is flowing through your body. Energetic flow is a *precursor* to biochemical activity. Naturopathy (as a philosophy), on the other hand, is more concerned about the biochemical imbalances that may be occurring in the body. Chiropractic seeks to correctly align the spine by mechanical adjustment, so that nerve signals flow properly—pinched nerves don't transmit information very well, and that can lead to health challenges or disease. All three healing systems are valid and very useful for overcoming ailments. If you can afford it, I suggest using all three disciplines, and letting your caregivers know that you are in counsel with other practitioners.

Here is an overview of some of the most popular and important therapies available. My ideal clinic would offer traditional Chinese medicine, naturopathy and chiropractic. The advantage of this is the "cross-knowledge" that the practitioners share by working closely with colleagues in different fields.

Traditional Chinese Medicine/Acupuncture
Nearly five thousand years ago the ancient Chinese recognized a vital energy behind all life forms and processes—this animating force controls the functioning of every organ and system in the body. The Chinese called this energy qi (pronounced chee). The Chinese word and character was originally "latinized" as "chi." Chi is known as the "life force" by shamans, as "prana" by yogis, as "bioelectric energy" by modern scientists, and the "vis medicatrix naturae" ("healing power of nature") by modern naturopathic physicians. This term, apparently coined by Hippocrates (a physician who lived 2400 years ago), shows that naturopathic medicine is deeply rooted in the origins of traditional Western medicine.

This life force energy must flow freely and in the correct strength and quality for the body to function correctly. In all illness, the flow of vital energy has been impaired, and the goal of traditional Chinese medicine/ acupuncture is to help restore the proper flow of energy (chi) throughout the body. Correcting an imbalance in energy flow is like fixing a template or blueprint—often preventing an impending illness before it can manifest physically. It's said that in ancient China people paid a doctor as long as they stayed healthy; if they became ill, payment was suspended until health was regained!

Healing practitioners discovered that chi flows along specific pathways, or channels, called "meridians." Each pathway is associated with a particular physiological system and internal organ. Disease arises due to a deficiency or imbalance

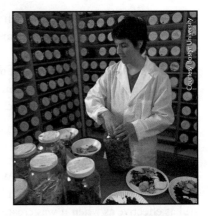

Chinese herbs are custom prepared for each patient.

of energy in the meridians and their associated physiological systems. TCM uses an intricate system of pulse and tongue diagnosis, stimulation or sedation of key points and meridians, a thorough medical history and detailed observation of symptoms to create a composite diagnosis. Two people with the same illness may have very different constitutions and causes for the condition. Therefore, an individualized treatment plan is formulated to assist each person in regaining a balanced state of health.

Chinese herbs are either ingested (often as a tea) or applied externally to balance body energy and revitalize cells and tissues. Acupuncture is the process of inserting very fine needles into precisely located points along the meridians with the intent to decrease, increase or shift the flow of chi. Modern science has measured the electrical charge at these points, corroborating the locations of meridians. Each point has a predictable effect upon the vital energy passing through it. According to the manipulation of the needles, energy can be drawn to a deficient organ, excess energy dispersed, blockages removed, and so on, according to the individual need of the patient. Acupuncture needles usually produce a slight stinging sensation, but rarely cause overt pain.

Sometimes points are treated with a special, heated herb—artemesia vulgaris latiflora (called "moxa")—which resembles a brown colored wool. Usually a small cone of moxa is placed on the skin over an acupuncture point, ignited, and removed when the heat is felt. Like needles, moxa revitalizes, reinforces, invigorates and restores balance and harmony to the vital energy.

As the balance and harmony of the vital energy is restored, symptoms of illness disappear. If all organs and functions of the body are working properly and harmoniously, there cannot be sickness within the body or mind.

Ayurveda

Known as "The Science of Life," Ayurveda is a Sanskrit word that literally means "life wisdom." Practiced in India at least 5,000 years ago (and still as effective as when it was created by ancient sages known as Rishis), Ayurveda is a natural system of medicine that employs diet, herbs, cleansing and purification practices as well as yoga to effect healing. The Rishis—masters of meditation and observation—developed a system of healing based on the five basic elements: ether, air, fire, water and earth. Combinations of these elements are known as the doshas. Your dosha is your constitutional makeup. There are three main types, called Vata (predominately air) Pitta (predominately fire) and Kapha (predominately earth and water), and four combination types. By knowing your type, you have immediate access to useful information on what to eat, how to exercise, how to cleanse and purify your body and how to prevent disease. Many natural food stores carry specific products, such as teas, which have been developed for the various doshas. Generally, you visit an Ayvuredic physician to have a complete profile and healing system created.

Naturopathy

Naturopathic medicine is a system of natural healing deeply rooted in Western culture. It is based on a philosophy that health and disease are on a continuum, and that the body has a profound ability to heal itself when given the proper conditions. Therefore, naturopathic patients are taught how to access the body's innate wisdom, promote vibrant health and prevent disease. Preventive care results in financial benefits, as health is maintained, disease avoided, and costly procedures averted.

Naturopathic physicians (NDs) treat 'the whole person,' taking into account the body-mind-spirit interconnection and the individual needs of the patient. Spending up to 90 minutes for an initial visit and an average of 45 minutes for follow-up exams, the naturopath asks numerous questions, performs a detailed physical exam, thoroughly investigates symptoms and complaints, explains treatment options and includes the patient in choosing a treatment plan.

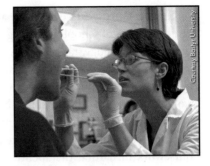

Naturopathic physicians are primary care providers (family physicians) and, like a conventional doctor, an ND will often use a number of laboratory procedures as well as the physical exam to make a diagnosis. Additionally, nutritional status, metabolic function, and toxic load are frequently considered to aid in diagnosis and treatment decisions. Non-invasive therapies such as lifestyle or behavior modification and relaxation techniques may be "prescribed."

Spinal manipulation, massage therapy, therapeutic nutrition, botanical medicine, detoxification, physiotherapy, exercise therapy, homeopathy, acupuncture and psychological counseling may also be included in treatment. In some states where naturopathic physicians are licensed, naturopaths may also perform minor outpatient surgery and prescribe medication. When prudent, an ND will refer patients to a specialist for a definitive diagnosis and advice.

Though naturopathy came to the United States just over 100 years ago, the natural therapies and the philosophy on which it is based have been effectively used to treat diseases for thousands of years. In fact, the word physician comes from the Greek root meaning nature. Hippocrates coined the phrase, "nature is the healer of all diseases." This concept underlies the principles outlined in the "Hippocratic Oath," as stated below:

- First, do no harm.
- Act in cooperation with the Healing Power of Nature (the 'vis medicatrix naturae' in Latin).
- Address the fundamental causes of disease.
- Heal the whole person through individualized treatment.
- Teach the principles of healthy living and preventive medicine.

The first two years of naturopathic school are very similar to conventional medical school, requiring anatomy, physiology, pathology, biochemistry, neurology, radiology, minor surgery, microbiology, obstetrics, immunology, gynecology, pharmacology, pediatrics, dermatology, clinical laboratory and physical diagnosis, among other courses. The second two years focus on clinical skills: NDs receive training in a wide range of natural therapeutics such as botanical medicine, homeopathy, natural childbirth, acupuncture, physiotherapy, and clinical nutrition. Because coursework in natural therapeutics is added to a standard medical curriculum, naturopathic doctors receive significantly more hours of classroom education in these areas than do graduates of many leading medical schools. Students also complete a clinical internship consisting of 1,500 hours treating patients under the supervision of licensed naturopathic and conventional medical physicians in an outpatient setting.

Currently, naturopathic physicians are licensed as primary care providers in 13 states and several territories, including the District of Columbia and Puerto Rico. Several provinces of Canada have licensed naturopathic physicians. England, Australia, and New Zealand also have provisions for appropriately trained naturopaths to practice.

It is important to recognize that in jurisdictions that do not license naturopathic physicians, anyone can refer to themselves as a naturopath or naturopathic doctor. While these practitioners, some of whom have been educated by distance learning, may have good information about natural healing, they may not have the training to recognize when to refer, nor have the knowledge to work in a complementary fashion with conventional health care providers. To find a qualified naturopath, visit the American Association of Naturopathic Physician's Web site at www.naturopathic.org and chose a naturopath from their database.

Homeopathy

[Note: Naturopaths are trained in homeopathy, but not all Homeopathic practitioners are Naturopaths.]

Homeopathy was developed by German physician and chemist Dr. Samuel Hahnemann in the early 1800s. Through numerous experiments, he furthered the theory of "The Law of Similars," that a substance in small doses can alleviate symptoms similar to those it causes at higher doses.

He believed that the microdose of a substance would stimulate the body's immune system to heal whatever pattern of symptoms would be found in a large dose of the same substance. This principle is also known as "likes cure likes," one of the two cornerstones of homeopathy.

Homeopathic remedies are prepared by a detailed process of repeated dilution and shaking, which makes them capable of stimulating the body's own defense system. The shaking, or "succussion," is the second cornerstone of homeopathy. Hahnemann believed that dilution and succussion released a power that affected the life force energy at the subtle (spiritual or energetic) level. For example, we are all familiar with formerly invisible, immeasurable, unknowable energy forms, such as electromagnetic radiation and subatomic particles. Magnets exerted their force long before science could explain the mechanism. Physicists are still trying to explain gravity and the nature of matter, still discovering phenomena such as the *strong force* and the *weak force*. Similarly, homeopathic medicine works at a level not entirely recognized by some in modern allopathic medical science.

Homeopaths believe that although the physical molecules of the original substance may be gone, dilution and succussion leaves something behind—an imprint of its essence, or its *energy pattern*—that gives it a kind of healing charge. Scientists who accept the potential benefits of homeopathy suggest several theories to explain how the highly diluted remedies may act. Using recent developments in quantum physics, they have proposed that electromagnetic energy in the medicines may interact with the body on some level.

Homeopathy is not yet well known in the United States, but is gaining popularity because of its high success rate in helping people, especially those who cannot be helped by conventional medicine. Homeopathy is very well-established and respected in England, France, Switzerland, Germany, India and many other countries.

In most cases, homeopaths consider everything that is going on in the patient's life rather than looking at isolated symptoms. The patient complaining of headaches may also suffer from depression, insecurity, low energy and a long list of other problems. All of these problems may stem from the same root cause; if so, then by dealing with the root cause, all of the problems will fade away. During a lengthy initial appointment (usually about 90 minutes) all of the complaints will be explored. Then the appropriate remedies, made from plants, minerals and other natural substances, are prescribed. Sometimes the remedy is given in a single dose and allowed to work over a period of time. In other instances, an initial dose is given, followed by repeated doses over a period of hours, days or weeks.

Homeopathy is often effective with people who have chronic diseases, long-term physical or emotional problems or recurring illnesses. After taking the correct homeopathic remedy, patients feel greater well-being and happiness, since homeopathic care goes much deeper than most other treatments. Whether or not conventional medicine considers the condition curable is *not* the major factor in determining whether homeopathy can help. Homeopaths recognize the importance of intervening as little as possible. They know the body is intelligent and produces symptoms for a reason.

Use of homeopathic remedies can never harm the body. Even if they don't work, they will not hurt. An experienced practitioner can help you use them in a way that won't spoil the curative action of the potencies.

Classic Chiropractic

Chiropractic care began with D.D. Palmer in 1895 when a janitor, who had been deaf in one ear, was able to hear again once Palmer pushed one of his vertebra back into place. The janitor had a vertebral subluxation in his neck, meaning the vertebra was stuck in an abnormal position. Palmer moved the vertebra back into position, and when he did, nerves in that region were able to function again, restoring the janitor's hearing.

Palmer realized that when misaligned vertebrae are physically adjusted into proper alignment, nerves supplying the afflicted region then operate at greater efficiency, allowing the body to more fully heal itself. Conversely, when vertebrae remain misaligned, the nervous system is compromised, and many parts of the body are not able to function optimally, which can lead to functional problems or disease. Chiropractic care is the process of physically aligning vertebrae back into appropriate positions so that nerve signal flow is restored to full function.

Network Spinal Analysis

A number of years ago, Dr. Donald Epstein, a chiropractor in New York, noticed that many chiropractors used techniques that encouraged the spine and nervous system to realign *on its own* via gentle stimulation, as

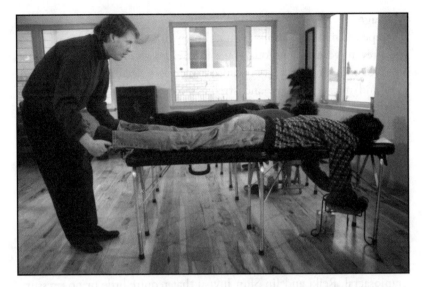

Network Spinal Analysis helps to stimulate the body to automatically realign the vertebra. I had great success from the above practitioner.

opposed to traditional physical adjustments. Some techniques worked around the neck area, others near the tailbone, and still others at specific vertebrae. Each method was aimed at getting the spine and nervous system to realign without physical manipulations. He discovered that these methods achieved excellent results and, after a great deal of research and testing on his own clients, developed network spinal analysis, a synthesis of effective low-force adjustments. Network spinal analysis uses gentle touches to the spine and meninges (tissue around the spinal cord) to stimulate the nervous system and spine to properly align.

Of particular interest is the "respiratory wave," which, when it flows through the spinal system, indicates that the system is realigning itself to optimal functioning. When the nervous system is operating without interference—whether from a subluxated vertebra or tension on the nervous system from the spine in another form—then the body can achieve a higher level of healing. Many people report that symptoms of headaches or other complaints disappear after a series of Network adjustments. I personally benefited greatly after receiving numerous treatments from two caregivers.

Massage

Therapeutic massage, also known as bodywork, is one of the most pleasant preventive care methods you can use. Its various forms have been used for thousands of years because it increases circulation, relieves tension and muscle spasms, and stretches connective tissue. It can break down or prevent the formation of adhesions, reducing the risk of fibrosis, and can actually increase the number of red blood cells, especially in cases of anemia. Massage improves muscle tone and can prevent or delay atrophy resulting from forced inactivity. It also stimulates lymph circulation and assists the elimination of wastes, lactic acid and other toxins.

There are many kinds of massage available, from direct intervention techniques like Rolfing (connective tissue restructuring named after founder Ida Rolf) and Swedish massage, to modalities like Shiatsu, acupuncture and reflexology, which act by releasing energy through the connective tissue. There are also "full on" energetic modalities such as craniosacral, Reiki and Jin Shin Juytsu that require little or no pressure. On the other hand, neuro-muscular therapy (NMT) and myofascial release are techniques that utilize a significant amount of pressure and can be somewhat uncomfortable (that "good hurt" feeling) during treatment, but provide pain relief after the session. Still other types of bodywork, such as Rosen, Rubenfeld and Hellerwork (all named after their founders) focus on emotional release. There are dozens of other choices, from Watsu (sessions conducted in the water) to the patented "BodyTalk," as well as sports, Russian and Thai medical massage. Still others offer what's known as somatic education. These modalities offer postural awareness and movement reeducation along with "tablework." They include Trager, Feldenkrais and Hanna Somatics (again, the disciplines bear their founders' names).

Thomas Claire's book, *Bodywork*[8] is an excellent reference that provides an overview of many kinds of touch therapies and takes you through the author's experience of each one. It also gives contraindications (conditions you may have which should not be addressed by massage therapy), explains the training regimen and gives reference phone numbers for each discipline, so you can call for recommended practitioners in your area.

Once you know the kind of work you're looking for, check the Yellow Pages and pick up some business cards from local bulletin boards. Call a few therapists and ask whether she is nationally certified and how long she has been in practice. Much of your experience will depend on the connection you feel with the therapist. Bodywork/massage is a burgeoning field and there are some people in it just for the money (even though it is hard work)! Look for someone you sense has a true dedication to facilitating healing through touch, and a commitment to excellence and continuing education. Glance at the certificates that should be displayed in the office and notice whether professional ethics are posted.

By the way, while an office in a clinic or sports facility may feel more professional, it's also very common and legitimate for a therapist to work from a home office, or even to give you a massage in your own home! Regardless of where your session occurs, you should feel comfortable at all times. Sheets and towels should appear clean and freshly changed.

While massage therapy isn't cheap (session rates vary across the country, but usually range between $45 and $85 an hour), it's less than most other medical professionals charge for a much shorter visit. And you'll save money in the long run.

Natural Medicine Conclusion

I hope you've gotten a sense of the exciting possibility of participating in your wellness. As Dr. Candace Pert, former head of the National Institutes of Health states: "We have far more control over our bodies and our health (or disease processes and their outcomes) than we realize." It's true. We need to re-empower ourselves by learning to listen to the wisdom of our bodies, and use healthcare professionals as partners rather than looking to them to provide all of our answers.

Natural Remedies

There are many natural remedies, found in natural food stores, that you can use. In addition to homeopathic remedies, which are discussed in detail earlier in this chapter, the three primary natural healing remedies you'll find in natural foods stores are: 1) flower remedies, 2) essential oils (aromatherapy), and 3) herbs/herbal combinations. Of course there are others, but these are the main categories (as opposed to "supplements," which are discussed in Chapter 6). For emotional issues, trauma and personality challenges, look into homeopathy, flower essences and aromatherapy. For overall well being, consider herbs and aromatherapy. For

ailments, try homeopathy and herbs, then flower essences and aromatherapy. To assist in your choice, talk with natural food store employees,
visit a natural doctor and/or read one of the books listed at the end of
this chapter.

Flower Remedies

Flower remedies are carefully prepared diluted essences of plants and
flowers that work on what's known as the subtle energy body as well as on
the emotional body. This means they work with the body on an energetic
and emotional level rather than a directly physical level. Dr. Edward Bach
(1897-1936) developed the first system of flower remedies, called the
Bach Flower Remedies. He believed that physical problems were mani-
festations of emotional problems, and that if the emotional problems
could be healed, that the physical problems would also be healed. Bach
discovered that certain flowers and plants stimulated the body's natural healing systems and helped to stabilize emotional problems. Whereas
Homeopathic remedies stimulate a polar opposite response in the subtle
energies, Flower Essences do the reverse and "pull" the subtle energies
into the direction of healing (wholeness).

In an interview with Better Nutrition, David Vennells, author of *Bach
Flower Remedies for Beginners*, Vennells explains that flower remedies are
a safe and gentle practice. "Flower essences can be used by anyone," he
writes. "They are generally prescribed according to our personality type
or the prevailing state of mind during a particular illness."

"Dr. Bach found a way to harness the healing energy contained
within certain plants and trees," said Vermeils. He explains how flower
essences work: "All living things possess life force energy. In the East this
is sometimes called chi or prana. It is a subtle type of life-giving energy.
Some plants and trees carry a particular type of life force energy which
can have a healing effect on the body and mind. Flower essences capture
and hold this healing life force energy until it is needed." To help treat an
illness, the appropriate flower remedy is prescribed by considering mental and emotional symptoms, rather than physical ones.

According to Vennells, flower essences help patients regain good
health or manage difficulties with a more positive attitude. He stressed,
however, that you don't need to be sick to reap the benefits of flower essences. "You don't have to be ill," he said. "They can just make life a lot

more meaningful. Although we may generally feel physically and mentally okay, we might also occasionally feel something is missing from our life, some meaning or purpose. This subtle feeling is a gentle wake-up call."

Essential Oil Aromatherapy

Ever smell a flower and feel better? You just experienced Aromatherapy! "Aroma," of course, means "smell or fragrance" and "therapy" means "treatment." Unlike the senses of sight, hearing and taste, our olfactory (sense of smell) nerves are connected directly to the brain. The sense of smell registers in the hypothalamus gland, which regulates many important activities, including those of the endocrine system, which controls hormones that affect growth and autonomic processes such as heart rate, breathing, digestion and body temperature. Aromatherapy uses pure, non-synthetic essential oils extracted from many parts of a plant (flower, leaf, resin, bark, root, seed, berry, etc.) to relax, balance and rejuvenate the body, mind and spirit.

In Aromatherapy, the essential oil is often diffused into the air or placed directly onto the body in a diluted base of oil or water. Most natural food and herb stores carry essential oils. Organic oils are the best. This safe and effective natural remedy helps to stimulate emotional balance in a delightful way!

Herbs

The use of healing herbs dates back tens of thousands of years. When used *properly and with care*, they are generally quite safe, while side effects, if any, are mild. (Specifically, I'm referring to pre-packaged medicinal herbs that include directions for their use; I'm not referring to the use of unpackaged bulk herbs used by the novice.) Medicinal herbs have the ability to work on specific systems of the body. Dozens of herbs and herbal combinations (called formulas) are available today to help facilitate healing in almost any area of the body. Choosing organically grown, wild-crafted herbs is always preferred. Purists believe that using the whole herb—not just a standardized extract from an herb—will give the best results.

Some herbs are considered tonics: nourishing specific cells, tissues and organs, and are often used for long periods of time. Tonics are very gentle, slow stimulants, and they provide nutrients that the body can use, such as vitamins, minerals, and many other properties, like plant pigments such as anthocyanins or flavonoids.

Other herbs are called specifics, because they have a specific job to do for a limited time (up to three 10-day cycles is common). They fine-tune biochemical processes, enhance the flow of chi and regulate energy in the bioenergetic channels (removing stagnancy and redistributing excess energy). They generally work by stimulating a process; one of the best examples is Echinacea, which stimulates immune cell function, heightening resistance to infections.

Still other herbs are called "heroics" (forcing remedies), as they blast through energy blocks and dramatically move or inhibit energy in the bioenergetic channels. They can be helpful when someone with a generally sound constitution suffers from severely imbalanced energies, and they should be used only by professional practitioners with knowledge of the herb's action and its contraindications.

Herbs are sometimes manufactured into tinctures, teas or capsules. Tinctures are either alcohol- based or glycerin (sugar) based. Tinctures are especially useful because they separate the active ingredients of the herb for easy assimilation and can be stored for long periods of time. Tinctures are stronger than teas and are frequently diluted in water. Teas work because when the herbs are heated, the active ingredients are released into the tea water. Some herbs work better as a tincture, others as a tea; still others are best raw (capsules). I suggest you always buy organic herbs, because in addition to being free of herbicides and irradiation, they will be more potent.

Vitamins & Minerals

Although vitamins and minerals can be considered natural remedies, I consider them to be supplements, since these nutrients ought to be part of your regular diet. If a deficiency is suspected, I suggest avoiding synthetic vitamins and minerals that are packaged as isolated units. Instead, take whole food supplements such as wheat grass juice or some of the other supplements I suggested earlier (see Chapter 6). Some herbs are high in specific minerals or vitamins, and that would be a good choice as well. Be as natural and as close to a living plant as possible. Isolated vitamins and minerals, even if found in a natural foods store, have been manufactured in a lab and should be used only if a better choice is unavailable.

Reference Books for Natural Remedies

If you desire to learn which natural remedies can help overcome specific ailments, I highly recommend the following books:

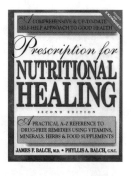

1. Prescription for Nutritional Healing by James F. Balch, M.D. & Phyllis A. Balch, C.N.C. Well-researched and very detailed, this best-selling book is an excellent resource which gives numerous natural treatment protocols for ailments from A to Z and is available in most natural food stores.

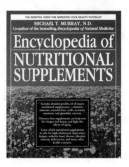

2. Encyclopedia of Nutritional Supplements by Michael Murray, N.D. Mr. Murray does a superb job of describing the various nutrients we require and why, and what happens when we don't get adequate amounts. He provides information on a number of natural remedies, as well as treatment plans for ailments. His work is very detailed and well-researched.

11
Dentistry
Go Holistic, for a Safe Smile

Nothing says "health" better than a vibrant smile. If you've got one, it's an asset you want to protect. If yours is less than perfect, you may want to take advantage of the advances in cosmetic dentistry to improve the appearance of your teeth. Actually, it's often more than just appearance: the state of your mouth affects your overall health. It's now well known that periodontal disease can cause heart problems,[1] and the American Academy of Biological Dentistry acknowledges findings that each tooth relates to a specific acupuncture meridian.[2] A misaligned bite affects chewing and digestion, and temperomandibular (TMJ) dysfunction can indicate other musculoskeletal problems. In this chapter, we'll discuss holistic dentistry, including fillings, root canals, fluoride use and periodontal disease treatment.

Holistic Dentistry Overview
Like their naturopathic counterparts, holistic dentists (also known as "bio-compatible," "biological" or "natural" dentists) consider the whole person (body, mind and spirit) and his or her lifestyle when recommending treatment. They understand the importance of a healthy immune system, and utilize treatment methods that will enhance overall health and wellness. Such dentists receive the same training as their conventional counterparts, and perform the same procedures. However, they minimize the use of x-rays (and/or use technology that reduces exposure

by up to 90%), and use non-toxic materials such as composite resins rather than mercury amalgam to fill cavities. Likewise, they address root canals and periodontal disease in a holistic, non-toxic manner. Services may include removal of amalgam fillings and detoxification of residual mercury deposits. Holistic dentists often work in conjunction with other complementary health care professionals.

Mercury Amalgam Fillings

The use of mercury in conventional dentistry is a serious controversy, and is probably the main reason to choose a holistic dentist—holistic dentists don't use mercury amalgam. Mercury amalgam ("silver") fillings contain about 50% mercury, a substance more toxic than lead, cadmium or arsenic. Traditional dental authorities allege that mercury is locked into the filling, because the atomic structure of mercury is "bound" to the silver, and therefore the mercury is biologically inactive. However, recent studies conducted at the University of Alberta, Canada show that mercury vapor actually escapes and is absorbed by the rest of the body. This increases when eating or drinking hot foods and liquids, during chewing (friction releases the vapor) or when placement of an amalgam filling is next to a tooth that has been restored with gold or other metals.

Mercury released from amalgam fillings has been shown to accumulate in organs, in fetal tissue and in maternal milk. This low-level (but continuous) mercury exposure may contribute to a variety of health problems if the immune system is compromised. Studies in animals and humans have shown decreased kidney function and an increase in antibiotic-resistant bacteria in the intestines. This low-level of exposure in experimental settings causes virtually the identical neurological alteration and degeneration of brain cells found in Alzheimer's Disease. For an excellent review of some of the compelling scientific research on amalgam mercury, see "The Scientific Case Against Amalgam," available from the from the International Academy of Oral Medicine & Toxicology Web site www.iaomt.org.

"Silver" (mercury) amalgam fillings are a potential health risk for everyone, but are of particular concern for those who are chemically sensitive. If you have a number of amalgam fillings and/or your immune system isn't functioning optimally, you may feel symptoms like lethargy, blurred vision, dizziness, muscle aches, numbness, etc. Consider having your amalgams removed—not only are they potentially harmful, they're also unsightly. Natural-looking composites are healthier and more aesthetically pleasing.

Removing "Silver" Fillings and Mercury

If you decide to have amalgam fillings removed, choose an experienced holistic dentist who follows specific protocols for protecting you from mercury exposure during the removal process, who can assess the biocompatibility of alternative materials, and who can refer you to someone skilled in mercury detoxification. The organizations listed at the end of this chapter should be of assistance.

Though silver fillings have been used routinely for the past 150 years, dentists have always been advised to handle mercury amalgam with extreme care. Strict protocols protect the dental staff. Left over "scrap" amalgam is considered hazardous waste by the EPA, so it's stored in a sealed, leak-proof container and taken to a certified, licensed metal recycling bin. Think about this: if the substance shouldn't come into contact with a dentist's fingers, should it come into contact with the more tender, often compromised tissues of the mouth—or placed anywhere near the brain, whose base lies just one inch from the roof of the mouth?

Quack, Quack, Where's The Duck?

Those who practice holistic, mercury-free dentistry are often labeled "quacks." Some have been harassed, or have had their licenses challenged or even revoked. Originally, a "quack" was a dentist who used silver fillings (mercury was known as quicksilver in the United States, but "quacksilver" in Europe). In 1848, the American Society of Dental Surgeons required its members to pledge NOT to use mercury amalgam in filling material. When member dentists in New York City used mercury, they were suspended for "malpractice by using silver mercury fillings." According to Morton Walker, D.P.M. (author of *Elements of Danger* and 70 other books related to alternative health), the suspended fellows refused to give up their toxic ways because mercury offered an easily malleable, inexpen-

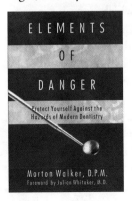

ELEMENTS
OF
DANGER
Protect Yourself Against the
Hazards of Modern Dentistry
Morton Walker, D.P.M.
Foreword by Julian Whitaker, M.D.

sive filling material. They formed a new, competitive organization—the American Dental Association!

Dental Mercury–An Environmental Hazard

In 1991, the World Health Organization convened a leading panel of experts in mercury toxicology to assess various sources of mercury exposure. They concluded that the single greatest source was *amalgam fillings*—greater than all other sources (food, fish, air and water) *combined*. Dental amalgams are no longer permitted in Sweden and may not be used during pregnancy in Germany, Austria and Canada, because the mercury goes directly into the fetus.

Another concern is municipal water contamination. Whenever an amalgam filling is placed or removed, the scrap amalgam (sludge in the form of very fine particles) gets scooped up by the dental vacuum unit and goes down the drain. Wastewater treatment agencies around the country have expressed growing concern about mercury levels in dental office wastewater, and many municipalities now require dental offices to be equipped with devices that capture and keep mercury out of the wastewater.

Root Canals

About the worst news you can get during a dental checkup is that you need a "root canal." (Most people would rather face an IRS audit than undergo a root canal!) Just what is this dreaded procedure?

Let's look at the anatomy of a tooth: Underneath the enamel on the surface of the crown (the portion of the tooth visible above the gums) is bone-like tissue called dentin. Dental pulp (which contains nerves, arteries, veins, and lymph vessels) lies inside the dentin. The pulp extends from a pulp chamber in the crown of the tooth to the tip of the root. This is the root canal. Although teeth can have more than one root (molars, for example, have two or three roots with canals in each root), all teeth have only one pulp chamber.

When the pulp is injured or diseased, your body will try to repair and heal it; if it can't, the pulp dies. This usually happens when bacteria invade the pulp chamber, either through a fractured tooth or a deep cavity, which can expose the pulp to the bacteria found in your own saliva. Supporting bone surrounding the tooth can be compromised or destroyed.

Root Canal Therapy

Root canal therapy involves drilling out the affected nerve and removing the pulp from the tooth. The pulp chamber and root canal(s) of the tooth are cleaned, sterilized, and sealed to prevent re-contamination. Although the treated tooth is no longer vital (it won't be able to sense pain, heat or cold), the natural structure of your mouth is retained, which is beneficial both structurally and aesthetically.

The procedure is controversial; some dental authorities estimate that as many as 80% of root canals are poorly done, often missing one or two roots. However, modern endodontists (root canal specialists) use computer-augmented x-rays and to find all of the roots and determine whether disease is present.

If you're considering a root canal, you probably have some apprehension, but the procedure is usually painless under local anesthesia. Some people worry that the tooth will fall out or turn black, but a restored tooth should last as long as other teeth because, as long as the root of the treated tooth is nourished by surrounding tissues, it will remain healthy. Discoloration is unlikely, but if appearance becomes a concern, the tooth can be bleached or veneered with porcelain or composite.

Now comes the controversy. Ideally, root canal therapy completely seals all of the canals associated with the affected tooth. However, after the nerve is drilled out, there are still several miles of microscopic tubules left and it's impossible to fill them all. Bacteria in these tubules can continue to survive, even after "successful" root canal therapy has been completed. Careful, sophisticated laboratory analysis has been done on root material from extracted root canal treated teeth, at Affinity Labeling Technologies, Inc.,[3] which has confirmed that significant bacterial toxins are present in many of these teeth. Presumably, these toxins can escape the porous root structure of the tooth and travel to other parts of the body. This has led many holistic oriented practitioners to recommend extraction as an alternative to root canal treatment, or to explore other alternatives.

Root Canal Alternatives

Injections next to the tooth with German isopathic remedies, procaine, homeopathics or ozone can sometimes save an infected tooth. Alternative treatments to root canals include extraction and thorough cleaning of the infected socket. If a root canal is required, then a particularly effective treatment is the use of a compound known as Endocal© (previously known as Biocalex©), which contains calcium oxide, zinc oxide and a special (ethyl/glycol/water) liquid that swells into the tubules, sealing them to prevent chronic infection.[4] The resulting substance, calcium hydroxide, has been repeatedly demonstrated to be the most biocompatible (safe) material available.[5]

Endocal© isn't used routinely in root canal therapy because its protocol is radically different from what is usually taught in dental school, where students learn to "compact" filling material into the canal to the greatest extent possible. Because of the volumetric expansion and penetration of calcium oxide, it has to be loosely compacted, allowing room for expansion to the apex of the tooth. Most endodontic specialists are skeptical of this concept, even though there's adequate science to substantiate it. If you can find a dentist or an endodontist who will use Endocal©, be sure it's noted on your records, because calcium hydroxide eventually converts to calcium carbonate and won't show up on x-rays, so a dentist you visit in the future won't be able to see that you've had a root canal!

The International Academy of Oral Medicine and Toxicology (IAOMT), considered by many to be a world leading authority on biological dentistry, has thoroughly investigated the root canal controversy in order to produce a "position paper" on this subject. They concluded that, at the present time, the available scientific evidence doesn't give a completely clear answer of "yes" or "no" about root canal treatment. Each individual case needs to be evaluated in the context of the whole person. That's really the core of a holistic dental practice.

And in my case, two weeks before completing this book, I decided to get a root canal treatment instead of an extraction for a tooth that was causing me grief. Interestingly, even though I was referred to an endodontist who uses Endocal, he suggested, and I agreed to, the use of the other filler: gutta percha. Further, I've been informed by a holistic dentist that Endocal© may contract after a couple of years, causing problems. So, please do additional research before making any decisions.

Periodontal Disease
If your gums are red, puffy or bleed easily when you floss, you may be one of the three out of four Americans over twenty with some form of

periodontal, or gum disease (some dentists think the figure is closer to 90%).[6] What is periodontal disease? The beginning stage is known as gingivitis, while the advanced stage is called periodontitis. To understand this serious, yet avoidable dental malady, let's look at how teeth are held in the mouth.

Teeth aren't embedded in the jawbones, but are totally surrounded by the periodontal membrane, a specialized tissue that acts as a shock absorber for the tooth. This membrane is actually a continuation of gum tissue that covers all of the bone in the mouth and all but the crown of each tooth. The periodontal membrane has thousands of tiny fibers called periodontal ligaments that attach teeth and bone. In a healthy mouth, there's a slight space between the tooth and the bone, called a pocket, which is usually about two to three millimeters deep.

Bacteria in the mouth like to collect into a sticky film called plaque, especially in protected areas like this two to three millimeters space under the gums. If this plaque isn't removed regularly (and effectively) with home care techniques, and if the body's resistance is low, then this bacterial plaque begins to overwhelm the immune system, and periodontal disease begins.

This can progress to create deeper pockets, and more infection, often with little or no symptoms that the patient is aware of. Periodontal disease can have other contributing factors such as stress, excessive pressure on a tooth caused by grinding, or from an asymmetrical bite. Excessive pressure on a tooth can also cause disintegration of the underlying bone. Poor fitting dental restorations can also be a factor, by causing the gum tissue around the restoration to become irritated.

For deeper, underlying reasons why periodontal infection can take hold, we have to look at imbalance in the body. TV commercials show how well certain mouthwashes kill the germs in your mouth, but don't mention that they'll be back within a few hours! The bacteria are part of a normal "population" that is always present. Disease isn't due to the presence of bacteria, but to the fact that they're breeding out of control, which causes inflammation. Effectively controlling the bacterial overgrowth is one part of treatment, but restoring balance in overall body chemistry and lowering stress levels is important for truly effective treatment.

High stress levels and poor diet lower immune system response and will deplete the body of many valuable vitamins and minerals needed for general maintenance and repair. If there's a shortage of calcium, phosphorus or other minerals, the body will take them from non-vital areas first (in this case, the jawbones) so vital organs can function. This weakens the bone supporting the teeth; subsequently, periodontal disease can be considered the beginning of osteoporosis.

Conventional Treatment for Periodontal Disease

Traditional treatment for periodontal disease involves surgical removal of the infected tissue and a course of antibiotics, sometimes administered by embedding a tetracycline-soaked chip or cord into the affected pockets. Surgery is painful and expensive, and there is often continued bleeding afterwards. Frequently, the surgery must be repeated within five years, because it removes the symptom rather than the cause. And while antibiotics can kill off weaker bacteria (and "good" immune building bacteria in the gut), the stronger bacteria become resistant.

Holistic Treatment For Periodontal Disease

A holistic dentist will use deep cleaning, teeth scaling and root planing to break up mats of bacteria and remove calcified tartar ("calculus") stuck to the teeth. Since a compromised immune system is recognized to be instrumental in the disease process, nutritional supplementation is a key aspect of treatment (decreased levels of vitamin C are associated with this disease).[7] The dentist will explain how the patient can brush, floss and "irrigate" teeth to effectively remove plaque and bacteria.

The patient's problem is there partly because old techniques and habits haven't worked well. New habits have to be learned and maintained. Many holistic dentists find that correct home use of an irrigating device (such as a WaterPik©) is one of the best forms of prevention, as well as an important adjunct to the periodontal treatment. Because the mouth has become overly acidic, a diet to restore the appropriate acid/alkaline balance is suggested (see chapter 5). The use of natural mouth rinses, such as "Ipsab," which contains prickly ash bark,[8] and the homeopathic remedies arnica, silicea and plantago greatly assist healing. In addition to Ipsab, many holistic dentists recommend MistOral, a topical gum spray, and The Natural Dentist Herbal Mouth and Gum Therapy oral rinse.[9] Other quality, natural products are becoming increasingly available at your local natural food store.

As the adage goes, prevention is the best medicine. Sugary, fluoride laden toothpastes and chemical mouthwashes have failed to protect the majority of us from gingivitis and periodontitis. Regular (and correct) brushing, flossing and irrigating with naturally compounded products and a healthy diet/lifestyle, along with professional treatment at appropriate intervals, should keep your smile healthy. Home/self care is an ongoing part of holistic dental therapy. Keeping gums healthy and resilient is not only mandatory for vibrant health, it's part of that all-important first impression smile that opens doors and gives you confidence both socially and professionally.

Fluoride and Fluoridation

Most of us have heard since childhood of the wondrous benefits of fluoride in toothpaste, drinking water and even supplements for infants. It might surprise you to learn that almost all holistic dentists are solidly against the use of fluoride and water fluoridation. They contend that the studies supporting the supposed benefits of fluoride are terribly flawed. A recent statistical look at decay levels in fluoridated versus non-fluoridated communities shows virtually no difference. Worse, fluoride is actually a very toxic substance and can cause harm at the same low doses that are recommended by water treatment authorities and public health officials.

I discuss the dangers of fluoride in Chapter 1. For a critical look at the fluoride issue, see www.fluoridealert.org or download the Position Paper on fluoridation from the IAOMT Web site (www.iaomt.org).

Conclusion

The practice of holistic dentistry is an integral part of complementary medicine. As we've seen, the mouth is an excellent barometer for systemic health. The condition of your teeth, gums and tongue are a window to the biochemical state of your body. Be sure to include regular dental exams in your health regimen, brush and floss at least twice a day and rinse with water after meals. Additionally, consider learning how to use an irrigator and buying a tongue scraper/brush. Your mouth will feel fresher and morning breath will be a thing of the past. Look for more "healthy" toothpastes and dental products at your local natural food store. As I said earlier, nothing says good health like a great smile—back it up with the confidence that yours reveals a healthy mouth that speaks for the whole body.

It's important to understand your options when it comes to choosing a dentist. Finding a good one is like finding a good car mechanic—they're both indispensable and worth their weight in gold. Contact the Holistic Dental Association at www.holisticdental.org or 970-259-1091, the American Academy of Biological Dentistry at www.biologicaldentistry. org or 813-659-5385, or the International Academy of Oral Medicine and Toxicology at www.iaomt.org or 863-420-6373 for informational pamphlets and recommendations in your area.

Dentist Recommendations
If you live in the Seattle area, I suggest visiting:
Dr. Mitch Marder or Dr. Paul Rubin
822-A NE Northgate Way
Seattle, WA 98125
206-367-6453

If you live in the Los Angeles area, I suggest visiting:
Dr. Raul Velazquez
11500 West Olympic Blvd., Ste. 335
Los Angeles, CA 90064
310-478-9393

Conclusion
You CAN Do It!

As you can see, the habits and lifestyles of contemporary culture will not lead us to vibrant health. Multinational corporations, the allopathic medical conglomerate, pharmaceutical empires, chemical companies, governmental agencies, advertisements, the meat and dairy industry, educational institutions and the mainstream media have homogenized into a self-perpetuating system that keeps us in the dark about the benefits of living a more natural lifestyle. So long as people are kept in ignorance—deliberately or not—the homogenized, synthetic culture that causes degenerative disease will prosper, at our expense. Yet, as we educate ourselves, educate others and apply natural living philosophies to daily living, the tide will turn and our collective health will be restored to full vibrancy, *as nature intended.*

Swimming against the tide of our synthetic contemporary culture—which, by the way, can include your friends, family and co-workers—is not always easy. But the best things in life are rarely easy to attain. Nevertheless, if I and millions of others can thrive in a natural lifestyle, so can you. Change can be intimidating or a bit scary, but by simply shopping at a natural foods store instead of at a conventional grocery store you're taking a huge step towards your goals. It's relatively easy, and once you've made the switch, everything else will follow.

By applying the principles of this book, you *will* be able to lose (or gain) weight, improve your energy, help prevent or reverse degenerative disease, increase your energy level, enhance your sense of well being and *attain vibrant health*. So, let's get started. Simply follow the steps listed in this overview to reach your health goals:

1. WATER: Make It Pure

Drinking pure water is essential to good health. As you learned in Chapter 1, most of our municipal water supplies include the harmful chemicals chlorine and fluoride, among other pollutants. Your best defense is to drink bottled water or use a high quality water filter that removes these toxins. The key is to ensure that chlorine and fluoride is removed, since most filters only remove chlorine. Reverse osmosis filters are high-end, but make sure the one you choose removes fluoride. My favorite filter is made by Custom Pure, and you can find their products at www.custompure.com. Also, consider using a chlorine filter on your showerhead, since we absorb more chlorine through the skin than we do through drinking water. The use of both filters will significantly reduce your exposure to harmful chemicals that have been proven to cause health problems.

2. FOOD: Friend & Foe

Most of our food supply is polluted with toxic chemicals and processed in ways that strip out much of the essential nutrition. In my opinion, the number one cause of degenerative disease is eating a constant diet of such non-nutritive food. The bottom line is that our bodies were designed to eat pure, "nature-made" food, not man-made synthetic food. We don't need to eat less food to lose weight ("dieting"); rather, we need to eat pure food (and we need to exercise) to lose weight. Most Americans overeat, and yet are malnourished. When we are malnourished, it's only natural to eat and eat and eat to try to get nutrition. Thus, stocking your home with only organic food is truly the way to go, no matter what the cost. Eating a variety of live, whole, organic foods on a regular basis is an essential step to follow if you want vibrant health. Organically grown food tastes better, is better for you and better for the environment; so give it a try and see what you think. I have an entire organic shopping list with suggested meal plans in the Appendix that you can use as a starting guide.

3. GROCERY SHOPPING: The Natural Way

There are thousands of companies that specialize in creating natural products; they endeavor to provide us with goods that are as close to nature as possible (e.g. still in their *original* state). These products cost more because, typically, they are more expensive to produce and expire more quickly. Yet, these products are often superior to their synthetic, chemically derived counterparts. Some conventional grocery stores carry natural products in special sections; natural foods stores generally carry these products exclusively. Consider going "all the way" and converting your entire household! That includes food, health and beauty aids, cleaning supplies and products made from recycled resources, such as bath tissue and paper towels. When you make this commitment, you, your family, pets and your home itself benefit from using non-toxic products.

4. SUPPLEMENTS: Daily For Vibrant Health

It would be great to get all our nutritional requirements from food. Unfortunately, even eating 100% organically grown food (which isn't easy to do) is unlikely to provide us with all our nutritional requirements because most soil is depleted of essential minerals. Thus, using whole food, nutrient-dense supplements on a daily basis is a great way to make up the difference. I suggest taking a super green food—such as spirulina, chlorella or Klamath Lake Algae—and probiotics, enzymes, flax oil and organic apple cider vinegar every day. Don't forget to try the seaweeds (such as dulce) which also have high concentrations of minerals from the sea salt (which can be found in the macrobiotic section). This daily mix will help fulfill your nutritional requirements. As you learn more, try other available options.

5. DETOX: Cleansing Is Essential

Detoxifying your body of harmful chemicals and biological pathogens is *absolutely essential* if you want optimum health. I can't stress this enough. Toxins that accumulate in the colon will at some point in time be moved to other parts of the body, and when that happens, the beginning stages of degenerative disease occur. Therefore, cleaning the colon on a regular basis is *mandatory* if you want to prevent or reverse degenerative disease. Cleansing the colon also improves digestion and assimilation of nutrients. Cleaning your colon is the first step to detoxifying your body, along with other modalities I've mentioned (such as drinking wheat grass juice) to remove toxins at a cellular level. I do a moderate three-day cleanse every three months and a full five-day cleanse twice a year. It's made all the difference in my life. You can follow the guidelines I give in Chapter 7, and/or consult a qualified health care professional such as a naturopathic doctor or a colon hydrotherapist. Again, detoxing your body is *absolutely essential* if you desire vibrant health—once you do it, you'll understand what I mean and you'll want to do it on a regular basis.

6. EXERCISE: For Confidence & Health

I started exercising four years ago and I wish I'd started 15 or 20 years ago. Regular exercise makes a huge difference in the way we feel and look. Every book I've read on financial success has included exercise as a necessary component. I believe it now. When I really push myself at the gym I feel more confident, have more energy and accomplish more during the day. The endorphins released during exercise really make a difference in my outlook, especially when facing multiple challenges. Exercising *vigorously* for at least 20 minutes a day is the minimum we need to make a difference. This is where your will power comes into play—you have to will yourself to find a gym (or outdoor exercise), and then get into an exercise routine. Trust me, you'll be much happier once you begin this routine. Not only will you feel better, but your health will improve, too. I belong to *24 Hour Fitness*, and I like the way their program is set up. I've heard great things about *Curves for Women*, and women may want to consider that club. In any event, the most important thing is to find an exercise routine and stick to it, because the benefits are too important to skip.

7. CHI ENERGY: Develop Your Personal Power

Developing your chi energy means developing your personal power. Your personal power is the part of you that is grounded, graceful and determined, *especially* when under pressure. When you are in touch with your personal power, you are less likely to react with fear and emotional outbursts when confronted with challenging words or actions. Instead, you'll be centered and graceful—yet determined—which will give you much greater respect among your family, friends, coworkers and peers. Yoga, tai chi and Aikido are great options for women; Kung Fu is an excellent choice for men. Although there are numerous health benefits associated with building your chi, I feel that the development of your personal power is probably the most important reason to pursue a chi building discipline.

8. DENTISTRY: Holistic, For A Safe Smile

It's amazing to me that one of the most poisonous metals in the world is used to fill cavities in our mouths. There is conclusive evidence that mercury vapor is released from amalgams fillings, and that some of the vapor is transmitted to and stored within cells. Simply put, that's low-level *mercury poisoning*, which can cause a host of health problems. In many states it is illegal for a dentist to tell clients this fact and the dentist can lose licensure for informing them (so much for the First Amendment guaranteeing free speech). The removal of this metal has improved the lives of many. Even though non-holistic dentists mean well, they are educated by an industry that promotes mercury amalgam fillings, and focuses on symptom management instead of on the holistic ecology of the mouth. By visiting a holistic dentist you improve your chances of regaining not only the health of your gums and teeth, but your whole body as well. Thus, for optimum health, visit a dentist who practices "mercury free" or "amalgam free" dentistry.

9. MEDICINE & HEALING: Battle Or Harmony

Perhaps the greatest tragedy in our modern times is that American culture has adopted a model of health care based on a reactionary system of disease management, rather than on one of preventive care and natural cure. Disease management with drugs and surgery is highly profitable; prevention of disease through education, and the reversing of disease through the use of highly effective natural, non-toxic medicine is not. Thus, we find a disturbing pattern of suppression of the knowledge of natural medicine within the allopathic (conventional) medical establishment, as well as the media. This needs to change if we are ever to regain our collective health. What's needed is a synthesis of the two modalities—allopathic and natural medicine—because allopathic medicine has amazing diagnostic tests to help uncover underlying conditions, and natural medicine gives us the understanding of how to correct those conditions. The bottom line is that natural medicine works. If you want to attain vibrant health, consider visiting a holistic doctor—such as a naturopathic physician—even if you feel great. Following the advice of a natural doctor will help ensure that you not only improve your health, but also prevent disease before it has a chance to begin.

10. VEGETARIANISM: High Fiber, Low Fat

Eating a strictly plant-based diet isn't that big a deal—except for people who eat meat. As a 14-year "veteran" vegan vegetarian,[1] the only comments I've heard about how I need to be concerned about my diet (or made fun of because of my diet choices) have been from meat eaters. Most such comments are just reiterations of meat and dairy industry propaganda rather than substantiated facts from their independent research into the topic. Despite the numerous comments I've heard from meat eaters, I'm a living testimonial—as are millions of other people—that eating a plant-based diet is a healthy option. So, if you feel that switching to a plant-based diet is right for you, then by all means, try it out. Just remember that all the rules of natural eating still apply: eat a variety of whole, live organic grains, legumes, vegetables and fruits on a regular basis. Some cities have local support groups, including the non-profit EarthSave foundation (www.earthsave.com), created by John Robbins. And if you feel that vegetarianism isn't for you, I encourage you to seriously consider eating only organic meat and dairy, so as to avoid pesticides, herbicides, artificial growth hormones, tranquilizers, antibiotics, preservatives and a host of harmful microorganisms. Organic dairy products made from goats' milk are much better for you and your family than dairy products made from cows' milk, as the protein profile of goat milk is similar to that of human milk.

11. APPPENDIX: My Shopping List & Meal Ideas

Following my shopping list and meal plans in the Appendix is a great way to get a jump-start into natural living. Perhaps the fastest and easiest way to take the next step is to start with a clean slate. If your budget allows it, throw away all your conventional foods, body care products and cleaning supplies and replace them with the products I include on my shopping list. Once you get the hang of buying natural products and making the meals I've outlined, you can experiment with the wide variety of high quality natural products offered today. Check my Web site for the DVD video I'll be producing which will take you on a step-by-step tour of exactly what to do to live the natural lifestyle. You'll catch on in no time, and I betcha you'll love it!

12. EDUCATION: Learn as you go

The Beginner's Guide to Natural Living is your starting point to natural living, and there is plenty more to learn to get firmly rooted in the natural living lifestyle. My Bibliography is an excellent reference for you because I have read some of the best books available on the subject. Another great place to continue your education is by browsing the book section of your local natural food store, and taking any of the classes offered at the store. My two all-time favorite books (for beginner's) are: *The Food Revolution* by John Robbins and *Cleanse and Purify Thyself* by Dr. Richard Anderson. Either book will help greatly as you move forward on the natural living path!

Appendix
My Personal Shopping List & Meals

When I explain the principles of eating natural foods, I'm often asked, "What should I eat?" I'm not a chef, and in fact I eat a very basic diet. Yet my meals are varied, nutritious and very delicious. Since you are probably new to the natural living lifestyle, you may wish to use my personal shopping list and meal suggestions until you are familiar with eating an organic, whole foods diet.

I have had the opportunity to help many people switch over to an organic diet, and I always begin by throwing away the food in their pantry and refrigerator that doesn't serve their health or well-being. I've heard the objection, "but I'm throwing away food—isn't that wrong?" My reply is, "Not when the food you are throwing away is detrimental to your health!"

Go through your pantry and fridge and toss everything that contains preservatives, additives, food dyes, or any other chemicals whatsoever. Just throw it away—it's not good for you or anyone else. (Do the same with all your body care products and cleaners as well!) Next, get rid of all the meat which is not organic—that stuff is packed with antibiotics, synthetic growth hormones, diseases and a host of other poisons you don't want in your body. Get rid of all your oils, sugar, margarine and iodized salt—they're not good for you either. When you are done, all you should have left are foods that don't contain added chemicals or unknown ingredients.

Now comes the fun part: go to the natural food store and start shopping for healthy food (and other items) for a better you! First I give a few shopping tips, and then my personal list of products I buy on a regular or semi-regular basis. I include the manufacturers so you'll be sure to buy products I know for a fact are of high quality. Even though I list quite a few products, it's very important for you to understand that I don't eat all of these food products all of the time.

For example, while I may eat fresh organic veggies from the produce section every day, I may eat chips or other snack food two or three times a month. Just because I list everything I use or sometimes use, that doesn't mean that each product has the same value to me. You'll get a much better understanding of what I mean when you read through my meal suggestions that follow the shopping list.

There are, of course, other products and brands to choose from that are equally excellent, so I encourage you to expand your buying patterns as you become familiar with the natural way of living.

Finally, it's very difficult to get fresh produce to look great in photography (especially in black and white!). There are photographers who specialize in nothing but food, and they hire "food stylists" to assist in the process. Thus, you'll find I don't include the fresh produce in the meal suggestion photography because it's simply too difficult to get good pictures of fresh food without spending a lot of money.

Natural Product Shopping Tips

Read Labels
Even when shopping at a natural food store it's important to read the labels. Get to know what's actually in the food you are eating. Since I'm vegetarian, I have found that a lot of food items contain animal ingredients, which I avoid. Try to avoid products that have added sugar, or any ingredients that don't seem right to you. If you don't know what an ingredient is, ask the store clerk for a definition, or choose another product.

Grains
I highly recommend grains such as brown rice, kamut, millet, quinoa and rye. To improve digestibility, soak grains for 6 to 8 hours, or overnight, and then cook them. Grains are excellent in stir frys, burritos and even soups. Stay away from white rice, since the nutritious brown layer has been removed.

Beans & Legumes
You can buy beans and legumes in bulk and save money over their canned counterparts, though it'll take you some time to prepare them. This plan may be desirable if you have a large family, because it's much less expensive. Soak dry beans and legumes overnight and simmer for two hours (or as per directions). They are an excellent source of protein.

Vegetarian
As you'll be able to figure out, my shopping list is a vegetarian list. It's easy enough to add meat or fish to any of my meal suggestions. If you eat meat, I suggest you choose only organic meat, because non-organic meat is highly contaminated.

Goals
As I mentioned earlier in the book, your goal is to eat organic, raw, whole foods as often as possible. Although there are a number of canned, boxed and refrigerated foods on this list, try to incorporate as much food from the fresh produce section as possible into each meal .

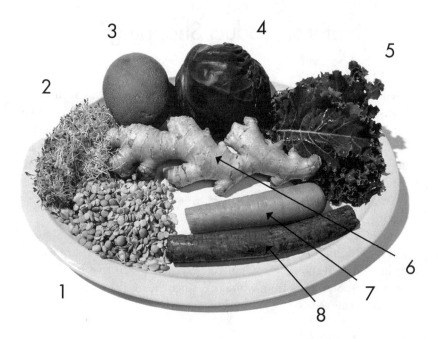

Fresh, Raw, <u>Organic</u> Produce

Eating whole, raw (uncooked), organic produce on a regular basis is essential to good health. Try to incorporate raw foods in every meal. It's okay to cook some produce, but it's also important to regularly eat raw produce because of the live enzymes and the "life force" that fresh produce contains. As I mention in Chapter 5, I also suggest you eat local produce, since it'll be the freshest and will have the proper energy (yin/yang balance) for your body. I explain how in the meal suggestion section.

1. **Sprouted lentils, peas, garbanzo beans, etc.**
   Why buy them canned or dried when you can get them freshly sprouted? Sprouted foods are *packed* with nutrition. Use them on salads, stir fries, burritos and other dishes. Of all the fresh foods available, these sprouted lentils, peas, garbanzo beans, etc. are some of my favorite because they are live, and so extremely easy to use in virtually any meal. Ask for them if you don't see them; they're often hiding.

2. **Crimson Sprouts**
Sprouts are delicious on salads and in sandwiches. Try alfalfa, clover, radish and the other varieties. Sprouts are full of live enzymes, which help with digestion. I like sprouts because they are so easy and quick to use: just grab and drop—no cutting and no fuss.

3. **Russet Potatoes**
I don't eat potatoes too often, but I do enjoy mashed potatoes (made with soy milk and Earth Balance Buttery Spread) and gravy (vegetarian) as well as stir fried potatoes with veggies and tofu. Yukon potatoes are my favorite. Try yams and sweet potatoes as well.

4. **Red Cabbage**
Red cabbage is great in cooked dishes, and lasts for a long time in the refrigerator.

5. **Kale**
Kale is an excellent "green" to eat because it is high in B vitamins. I cut the stem off and use just the leaf in cooked dishes.

6. **Ginger**
I add fresh ginger to most everything I cook. Ginger is a blood purifier and I love the flavor it imparts to my meals. Peel and grate.

7. **Carrots**
I add carrots to cooked dishes once in a while. However, where I enjoy carrots the most is as a fresh squeezed juice. *Organic* carrot juice is a powerhouse of nutrition, and has a very sweet flavor. Try it!

8. **Burdock Root**
Burdock root is a very grounding root vegetable, which makes it an excellent choice for vegetarians. It doesn't have much flavor, so I find it's best when cooked with other foods. I use it in soups. Peel the skin.

Not-Pictured
Avocado—excellent on all food.
Butternut squash—try it in soups.
Broccoli—delicious cooked, and quite nutritious.
Daikon radish—blood purifying radish that's great in cooked dishes.
Green onions—for salads.
Mixed greens—for salads.
Shiitake mushrooms—medicinal qualities; excellent in stir frys.
Tomatoes—for sandwiches.

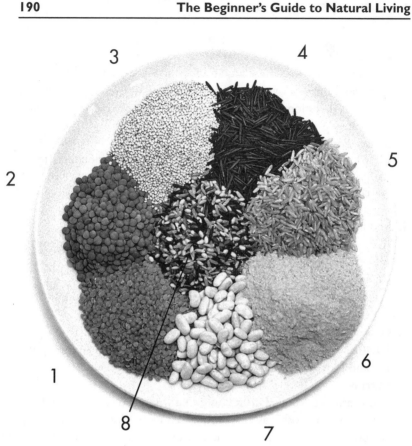

Organic on a Budget: Bulk Food

I often hear the objection, "But organic food costs too much." This claim simply isn't true. First, organic food is less expensive at natural food stores than conventional stores, so that's one of many reasons to shop at a natural food store. Second, if you are accustomed to eating primarily pre-packaged meals, then yes, organic could seem costly. Yet, if you create your own meals from scratch—such as I outline in my meal suggestions—then the cost drops dramatically. Finally, if you are feeding a large family, then buying grains, legumes, beans and other dried foods in bulk is certainly the way to go. The trick is to make these dried goods the "base" of your meals, and then add veggies and other foods (e.g. tempeh, nuts, beans, etc.) to that base. Everyone can afford to eat organic food when the priority shifts from pre-packaged meals to meals prepared from scratch.

There are a lot of grains to choose from at the natural food store, so you'll never get bored: quinoa, kamut, spelt, wheat berries, millet and many others. If you are a homemaker and manage a family, then rotating in a wide variety of grains (and other bulk foods) is an excellent way to save money and yet keep variety in your meals.

After I finished taking the photo on the opposite page, I dumped the contents into a pot of water, soaked it overnight, added sea salt, cooked it the next day, and used it for several days as a base that I mixed into my other foods. It was an delicious combination that worked with my meals.

1. **Red Lentils**
2. **Green Lentils**
   Probably the coolest thing about red and green lentils—besides their flavor and nutrition—is that they cook fast (20 minutes or so). Add to your soups, stir into stir frys or sprinkle on salads.
3. **Millet**
   Millet is one of those exotic grains like kamut, spelt, quinoa and others. There are many more grains than rice! Mix it up and you and your family won't get bored.
4. **Wild Rice**
   If you haven't tasted wild rice, then you are in for a treat. It has a distinct flavor that you'll appreciate.
5. **Brown Rice (long grain)**
   There are several varieties of brown rice to choose from. Basmati is very popular and tasty. Soak overnight to improve digestibility. Avoid white rice as it's been striped of its nutritious brown shell.
6. **Nutritional Yeast**
   Nutritional yeast is packed full of B vitamins, and adds a distinct flavor when sprinkled on salads, stir fries, burritos and similar types of dishes. I use it on my meals all the time.
7. **White Beans**
   White beans are really delicious and flavorful. Add to any soup.
8. **Rice Blend**
   You can even find mixed blends in the bulk section; great for variety.

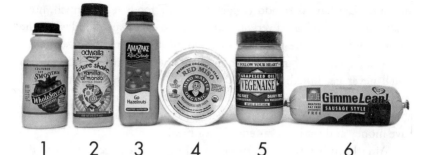

1   2   3   4   5   6

Refrigerator

1. Yogurt Drink—WholeSoy & Co.
A tasty non-dairy yogurt drink.

2. Soy Drink—Odwalla
I really enjoy Odwalla's "Vanilla Al'mondo" drink.

3. Rice Drink—Amazake
Delicious, all natural sweet rice drink.

4. Miso Paste (red or barely)—Master Miso
Since I love miso soup, I've tried several brands of miso paste. Master Miso is by far the best brand of miso paste available. Their chick pea miso is good for evening time. Their red miso paste is the one I use most often in the miso soup recipe (in the meal suggestion section). The red is nice because it dissolves quickly in hot water, whereas their country barley miso takes a little longer to dissolve (though it's an excellent choice as well). If you want great tasting miso soup, use Master Miso.

5. Mayonnaise (substitute)—Follow Your Heart
Vegenaise—Grapeseed version. There are a number of vegetarian mayonnaise substitutes that I've tried, and I like this one the best.

6. Sausage (vegetarian)—Lightlife
Gimme Lean—Tasty meat substitute. Add fried patties to any meal.

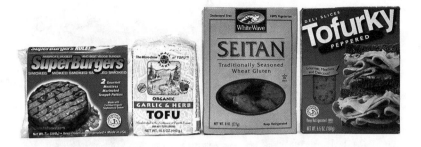

7   8   9   10

Refrigerator

7. Veggie Burger—Turtle Island
A delicious tempeh burger—tasty and filling. Highly recommended.

8. Tofu (Garlic & Herb)—Small Planet
If tofu is new to you, then start with the best tasting. Stir fry in oil and add shoyu or tamari sauce to taste. You'll be surprised how delicious it is.

9. Seitan (meat substitute)—Whitewave
A wheat glutton meat substitute that's often cooked like tofu. Once cooked, it's delicious in stir frys, burritos and on top of salads.

10. Deli "meat" (vegetarian)—Tofurky
The peppered version is nice; great for a quick sandwich.

NOT PICTURED
Buttery Spread—Earth Balance (organic)
The best non-hydrogenated dairy-free spread available; use instead of margarine or butter. Delicious on toast and other foods.

Ice-cream substitute—Soy Delicious
Vanilla flavor; the best soy "ice-cream" available (in the freezer section).

Burrito (vegetarian, organic)—Trader Joes (private label)
Found at Trader Joes, these burritos are delicious, filling and inexpensive.

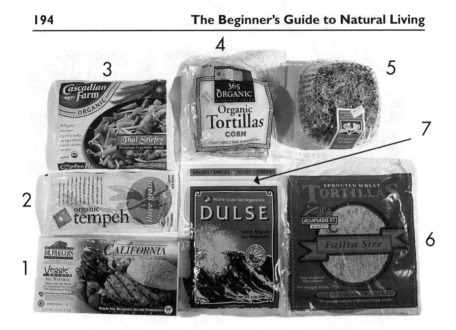

Refrigerator

1. Veggie Burger—Dr. Praeger's (*freezer section*)
Delicious "whole food" veggie burger that I really enjoy.

2. Tempeh (3 grain)—Lightlife
I prefer 3-grain variety. Stir fry in oil and add shoyu to taste. Very filling.

3. Vegetarian meals—Cascadian Farms (*freezer section*)
A variety of pre-made frozen meals—all are tasty.

4. Tortillas (corn)—365 Organic
Whole Foods natural food store private label. Inexpensive.

5. Sprouts—Local Vendor (*produce section*)
Try sprouted lentils, beans, nuts and grains as well. Sprouted food is very "alive" and packed with energy. Eat them as often as possible.

6. Tortillas (flour)—Alvarado Street
Large whole wheat flour tortillas that are great for burritos.

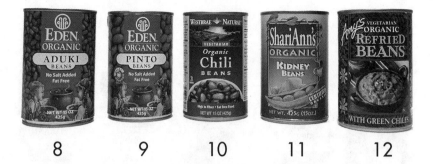

8　　　9　　　10　　　11　　　12

Dry Goods

7. Dulse Seaweed—Maine Coast Sea Vegetables
Especially good in soups, such as my miso soup recipe. A great source of vitamins and minerals. Find it in the macrobiotic section.

8. Aduki Beans—Eden
9. Pinto Beans—Eden
10. Chili Beans—Westbrae Natural
11. Kidney Beans—ShariAnn's
Canned beans
The only fresh beans you'll probably find at a natural food store are sprouted garbanzo beans (in the produce section), which leaves canned beans and dry beans as your primary bean options. Since I don't have a large family, I use canned beans. The great thing about canned beans is that they are nutritious, can be quickly added to most any cooked dish and they taste great. I often use *chili beans* for the variety, but I use the others as well. I think it is far better to whip up your own soup, chili or stir fry using fresh ingredients and canned beans than to eat fully prepared canned soups and meals. In fact, you won't find meals in a can listed in my book, because I don't eat them, and I don't find them nearly as tasty or nutritious as my own creations, in which I use canned beans as a primary ingredient. See my meal suggestions for how I use beans in my meals.

12. Refried Beans—Amy's
Vegetarian and organic: great for burritos. Heat in pot and add shoyu sauce and Mexican Spice seasoning (next page) to taste.

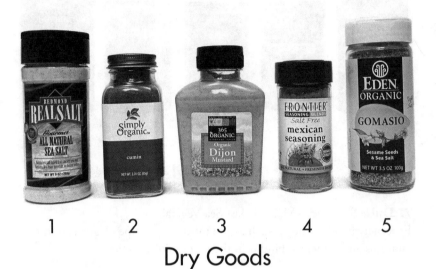

1   2   3   4   5

Dry Goods

1. Sea Salt—Real Salt
Sea salt is the only salt to use; Real Salt is a good choice for sea salt.

2. Cumin—Simply Organic
I use cumin quite a bit. Cumin blends well in burritos and stir frys, and is a spice that works with most foods. The flavor is unique. Try it.

3. Mustard—365 Organic
Whole Foods natural food store private label. For veggie burgers.

4. Mexican Seasoning—Frontier
I discovered Mexican Seasoning many years ago, and it's still my all time favorite spice. It's my first choice because it works so well with such a wide variety of foods. I never get tired of this spice and highly recommend using it in your cooked dishes, especially stir frys and burritos.

5. Gomasio Seasoning—Eden Organic
Gomasio is a sesame seed and sea salt blend that can be found in the macrobiotic section. Add this condiment to your finished dish.

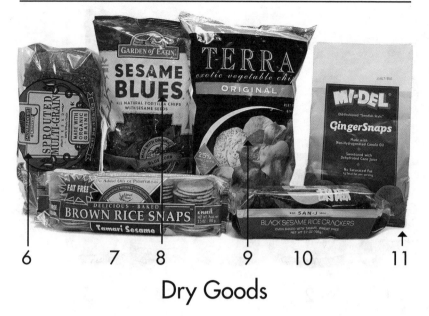

6 7 8 9 10 11

Dry Goods

6. Bread—Alvarado Bakery
Alvarado Bakery makes organic breads which are sold at most natural food stores, usually in the refrigerator or freezer section. I like their breads because they use sprouted grains and all natural ingredients. Check out your local organic bread bakery as well (in the bread section).

7. Tamari Sesame Crackers —Edward & Sons
Great with dips, such as hummus, and vegetarian deli "meats."

8. Sesame Blues chips—Garden of Eaten
All of their chips are excellent; I enjoy Sesame Blues.

9. Terra Chips—Terra Chips
Various root vegetable chips with a unique flavor; you must try them.

10. Black Sesame Crackers—SAN J
My favorite cracker. Very flavorful and filling. Pricey, but worth it.

11. Ginger Snap Cookies—Mi Del
These cookies are crunchy, delicious and addicting. Don't eat too many!

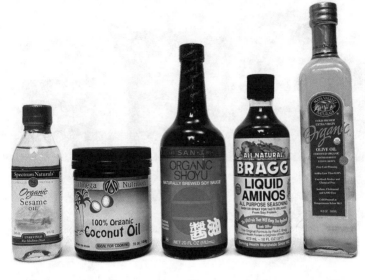

Dry Goods

1. Sesame Oil—Spectrum Naturals
Sesame oil is good for low temperature frying, and toasted sesame oil (not pictured) is excellent on pastas and salads.

2. Coconut Oil—Omega Nutrition
Coconut oil is great for all types of frying—minimal trans-fatty acids.

3. Shoyu (soy sauce)—SAN J
Shoyu and tamari (not pictured) are soy sauces, but aren't heavily processed like regular soy sauce. Shoyu is a salt replacer, and I use it in virtually all my cooking. Because it's a salt replacer, it's also quite grounding.

4. Liquid Aminos (seasoning)—Bragg
Liquid aminos is similar to shoyu, but it's processed differently and has its own unique flavor. I use liquid aminos when I'm not using shoyu.

5. Olive Oil—Napa Valley
This is my favorite olive oil. Good for salads and in cooked dishes.

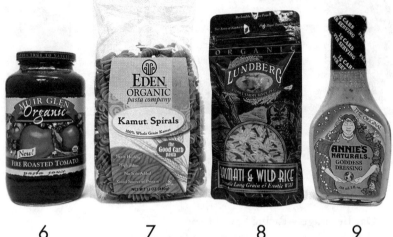

6   7   8   9

Dry Goods

6. Pasta Sauce—Muir Glen
Fire Roasted Tomato; pasta sauce for a quick, tasty meal.

7. Pasta—Eden
Kamut is a grain, just like wheat. Try something new!

8. Basmati & Wild Rice—Lundberg
A great rice combination for stir fries and other dishes.

9. Goddess Dressing—Annie's Naturals
I discovered Annie's Goddess Dressing many, many years ago. Since that time I have tried several other brands of dressings, but none have ever come close to tasting as good as Annie's Goddess Dressing. Whatever skill level you are as a cook, if you have Annie's Goddess Dressing on hand, you can make any dish taste great! They created the perfect flavor for all dishes, whether salad, stir fry, burrito or anything in-between. You must try it—it's really that good.

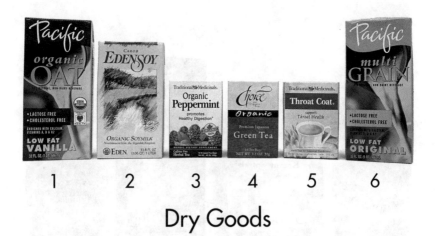

Dry Goods

1. Oat Beverage—Pacific Soy
Oat beverage is great as is, or on your favorite cereal.

2. Carob Soy Beverage—Edensoy
Carob is a delicious flavor that I recommend.

3. Peppermint Tea—Traditional Medicinals
A relaxing tea for the evening.

4. Green Tea—Choice
A light green tea that's good for the morning.

5. Throat Coat Tea—Traditional Medicinals
I use this when I have a sore throat and it works great.

6. Multi-grain Beverage—Pacific Soy
Multi-grain is my favorite beverage for cereals, and to drink as is.

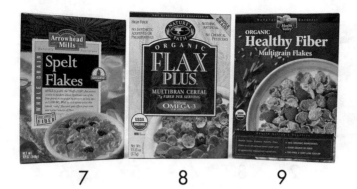

7   8   9

Dry Goods

7. **Spelt Flakes Cereal**—Arrowhead Mills
8. **Flax Plus Cereal**—Nature's Path
9. **Healthy Fiber Cereal**—Health Valley

Dry Cereals
As I mentioned in Chapter 5, I believe it's best if we eat whole, live food as often as possible, especially in the morning (such as my morning miso soup). Therefore, instead of eating cold cereal in the morning, which is a fairly yin (expanding) food, try eating it in the evening, which is a better time for a yin food. I never eat cold cereal in the morning, but from time to time I do eat all of the brands listed above, in the evening, often as a snack. I usually use one of the beverages on the previous page, and then add some organic almond butter and pure maple syrup. Sometimes I add berries. What a delicious evening snack!

Especially for Parents
Feeding children sugar laden cold cereal in the morning—day in and day out—can really cause a lot of problems with concentration in school, because sugary cereal is very yin (expanding—see Chapter 5). The miso soup recipe is an excellent alternative to cold cereal. Even hot cereal is better than cold cereal (because heated food is more yang–grounding). If you must feed your children cold cereal, then please switch to these healthy alternatives, and "sweeten" with almond butter instead of sugar.

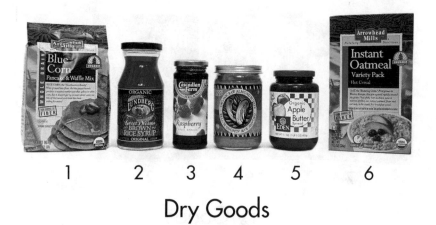

1   2   3   4   5   6

Dry Goods

1. Pancake Mix (blue corn)—Arrowhead Mills
Every now and then I enjoy eating pancakes, usually in the evening, since pancakes are a yin (expanding) food. I'm particularly fond of blue corn pancakes. Try adding fresh grated ginger to the batter for a delicious zing.

2. Brown rice syrup—Lundberg
A thick sweet syrup that has a butterscotch like flavor.

3. Raspberry fruit spread—Cascadian Farm
This raspberry fruit spread is my favorite.

4. Raw Organic Almond Butter—Trader Joes
I use almond butter in my miso soup (see the miso soup recipe) and sometimes in stir frys. Raw organic almond butter is expensive, though you can find it discounted at Trader Joes. The alternative is non-organic toasted almond butter, manufactured by Marantha (not pictured).

5. Apple Butter—Eden
This is a very tasty spread that doesn't have any added sugar. If you are trying to reduce your sugar intake, try this spread, because it's quite good.

6. Instant Oatmeal (variety pack)—Arrowhead Mills
A delicious cereal, hot or cold.

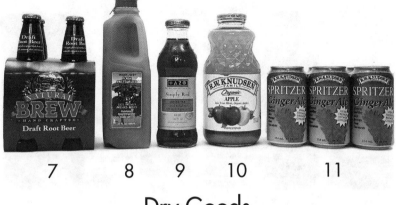

7   8   9   10   11

Dry Goods

7. Root beer soda pop—Smucker
All natural soda. Root beer is my favorite flavor.

8. Apple Juice (fresh–refrigerator)—Trader Joes
I'm addicted to fresh apple juice. I always have it in my fridge. I drink it straight and I add my drink powders to it (e.g. spirulina, wild blue green algae, hemp seed powder, etc.). Fresh apple juice is my all-time favorite drink, and I highly recommend it. Find it in the refrigerator section.

9. Juiced Tea (Simply Red)—TAZO
Juices and sodas may be too sweet for you or your children. However, TAZO makes several tea drinks which combine tea with fruit juice. These are very tasty alternatives to the much sweeter drinks available, and are great for you and your children. Hats off to TAZO for this product.

10. Apple Juice—R.W. Knudsen
R.W. Knudsen makes organic bottled juices, and their juices are far superior to the bottled juices you'll find in any conventional store.

11. Ginger soda pop—R.W. Knudsen
All natural soda.

Maple syrup (pure)—Spring Tree (*not pictured*)
Maple syrup is my favorite sweetener; use sparingly.

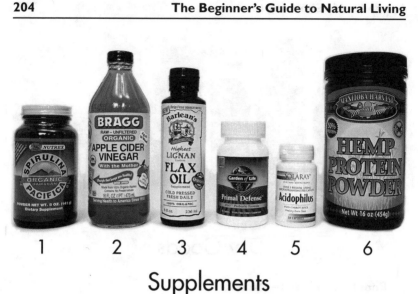

1   2   3   4   5   6

Supplements

1. Spirulina (Hawaiian, raw powder)—Nutrex
Mix heaping teaspoon with apple juice. Consume daily.

2. Apple Cider (organic)—Bragg
Only buy raw, organic apple cider vinegar that has the "mother."

3. Flax Oil—Barleans
Barleans and Omega Nutrition (not pictured) manufacture the best
tasting flax oil. I add flax oil to most of my meals, and prefer it over olive
oil. It's packed with essential omega-3 fatty acids, so I highly recommend
using flax oil every day. It's much better on food than by the spoon.

4. Primal Defense—Garden of Life
Friendly microorganisms for the intestines. Recommended.

5. Acidophilus—Solaray
Over 3 billion organisms per capsule for the intestines.

6. Hemp Protein Powder—Manitoba Harvest
Hemp seed is packed with nutrition and amino acids (protein), and you
can add this powder to your spirulina and apple juice combination.

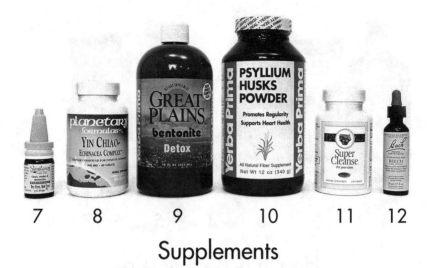

7   8   9   10   11   12

Supplements

7. Eye Drops (homeopathic)—Similasan
I use these drops when I wear contact lenses.

8. Yin Chiao Formula—Planetary Formulas
Yin Chiao is an excellent Chinese herbal formula for colds and flu.

9. Bentonite Clay—Yerba Prima
For colon cleansing (see Chapter 7).

10. Psyllium Husk—Yerba Prima
For colon cleansing (see Chapter 7).

11. Super Cleanse (herbs)—Nature's Secret
For colon cleansing (see Chapter 7).

12. Flower Essences—Bach
Choose the remedy based on your emotional state.

Colon Cleanse Kit—Arise & Shine (*not pictured*)
An excellent kit with virtually everything you need to get started. Pricey, but worth it! By Dr. Richard Anderson: www.ariseandshine.com

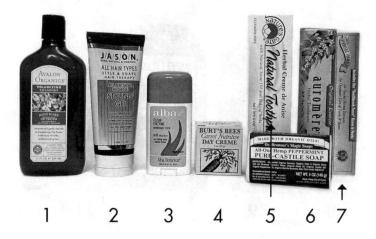

1   2   3   4   5   6 7

Health & Beauty Aids

1. Shampoo—Avalon Organics
I prefer their rosemary shampoo.

2. Styling Gel—Jason Natural Cosmetics
This is a great smelling and effective alternative to the chemical-based gels.

3. Deodorant Stick—Alba Natural Products
I use the Clear Enzyme aloe unscented. No aluminum or paraben.

4. Face Cream—Burt's Bees
Carrot Day Cream: A pure botanical cream (no synthetic chemicals) that helps to keep the face healthy.

5. Toothpaste—Nature's Gate
I prefer the Herbal Creme de Anise.

6. Bar Soap (peppermint)—Dr. Bronner's
Great all natural soap with essential oils.

7. Toothpaste—Auromere
Ayurveda toothpaste with neem and pelu.

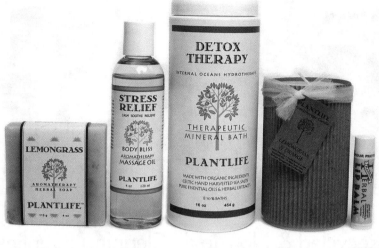

Pure Botanical Health & Beauty Aids

8. Aromatherapy Herbal Soap—Plantlife
A gentle and moisturizing soap for the skin. Contains pure essential oils, organic herbs and is infused with calendula and chamomile.

9. Massage Oil—Plantlife
Great for Massage, bath or just to put on your skin.

10. Bath Salts—Plantlife
These salts contain over 82 trace minerals (most salt on the market is washed and comes from polluted areas); some of the best available.

11. Aromatherapy Candles—Plantlife
Synthetic free candles made with plant-based waxes, pure essential oils and cotton wicks. They burn clean, contain no petrochemicals and smell great. An environmentally safe choice.

12. Lip Balm—Plantlife
Heals lips, cuts, bumps, cuticles and sores. No petroleum.

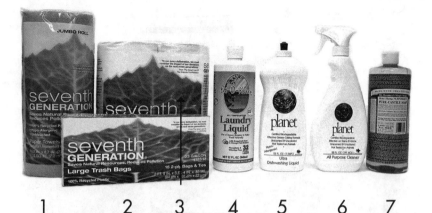

1   2   3   4   5   6   7

Recycled & Non-Toxic Cleaning Supplies

1. Paper Towels—Seventh Generation
Save trees, water and landfill space by using recycled paper products.

2. Trash Bags—Seventh Generation
Recycled plastic saves oil and landfill space.

3. Toilet Tissue—Seventh Generation
Works just the same as virgin toilet tissue, yet saves precious resources.

4. Laundry Detergent—Bio-O-Kleen
My favorite laundry detergent that cleans my clothes and makes them smell great (with a citrus smell).

5. Dishwashing Liquid—Planet
Gentle, non-irritating formula that effectively cleans dishes.

6. All Purpose Cleaner—Planet
Spray on, wipe off. Works great without toxic chemicals or fumes.

7. Pure-Castile Soap—Dr. Bronner's Soap
A peppermint body wash that doubles as an all purpose cleaner.

Detoxification Programs

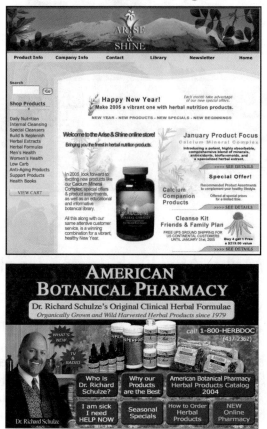

As you learned in Chapter 7, optimum health cannot be achieved unless you detoxify your body. Dr. Richard Anderson, of Arise and Shine, and Dr. Richard Schulze, of American Botanical Pharmacy, have created excellent cleansing programs, either of which I highly recommend. Dr. Anderson and Dr. Schulze share similar philosophies regarding colon health and diet, and have developed products especially for cleansing the colon. I recommend reviewing both of their programs.

www.ariseandshine.com and www.herbdoc.com

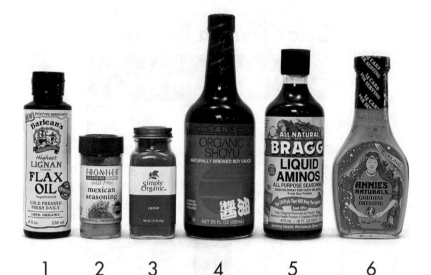

1　　　2　　　3　　　4　　　5　　　6

Make Any Dish Taste Great

My Secret Weapons
You don't have to be a chef to make quick, great tasting, all natural, organic meals. The key is proper seasoning and food combining. If you will stock the items listed on this page and use them as I suggest, you can't go wrong. I use these products all the time, I never get tired of them, and my friends and family always enjoy my meals. All you need to do is shift your cooking habits a little, and I think you'll find working with all organic, natural foods to be a wonderfully nutritious, tasty and uplifting experience.

1. Flax Oil

As I mentioned in the Supplements Chapter, flax oil is very high in essential Omega-3 and Omega-6 fatty acids, which is one reason to consume it on a daily basis. Well, it just so happens that it tastes pretty darn good when it's added to meals such as stir frys, baked potatoes, burritos and salads (right before the dish is served). Although I like olive oil, sometimes I find it to be too strong, whereas flax oil seems to have just the right strength of flavor. In fact, even though flax oil is sold as a supplement—which means drinking it in a tablespoon—I never take flax oil in that manner. I add it to my food instead. It's a flavor enhancer just like olive oil, only better tasting, in my opinion! Use it liberally on all your food and reap the benefits of the essential fatty acids and its flavor enhancing abilities. Keep refrigerated.

2. Mexican Seasoning

I add Frontier Mexican Seasoning to a lot of my cooked foods. It just has a nice punch that works with nearly every food combination. I never tire of this spice, but If I want variety, then instead I use:

3. Cumin

Cumin is also a great flavor that works well with many food combinations. I use it less than Mexican Seasoning, but I still use it a lot. A very distinctive flavor.

4. Shoyu Sauce

Shoyu sauce and tamari sauce are basically soy sauces, only they taste better and are better for you. Shoyu sauce is my <u>number one secret weapon</u>: it's a salt replacer that has way more flavor than salt (even sea salt). I use shoyu (or tamari) sauce in <u>virtually all cooked dishes</u>, to lesser or greater degrees. Think of it as your salt replacer. When you combine shoyu with cumin or Mexican Seasoning, you have an absolute winning combination that works with virtually all cooked foods. I never tire of this combination and I hope you try it—it's the best.

5. Liquid Aminos

This is similar to shoyu, only not fermented, with a "lighter" flavor. An excellent salt replacer as well. Plus, as the name suggests, this product is made of essential and non-essential amino acids—building blocks of protein—to help promote good health. Highly recommended.

6. Annie's Goddess Dressing

Add the world's best tasting salad dressing to virtually any dish and it will taste better—this dressing isn't just for salads! Use it on most cooked meals and you'll see how easy it is to make any meal taste better. I have yet to find a better tasting dressing than Annie's Goddess Dressing.

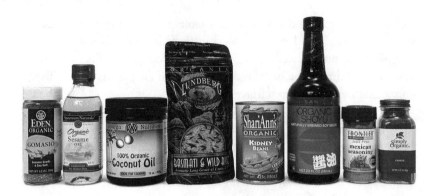

Stir Fry & Salad

Overview

The stir fry has an endless number of combinations, so you and your family will never get bored with this meal. Since the stir fry is cooked food, it's a good idea to add a salad so you get some "alive" food as well. Even the salad has plenty of food variations, making the stir fry and salad combination an excellent beginner's choice for you.

Stir Fry Preparation

Prior to beginning the stir fry, prepare your grains by soaking them overnight and then cooking them to completion. You can use brown rice, wild rice, kamut, wheat berries, quinoa, millet, rye or any other type of grain found in the bulk section or sold already packaged, such as Lundberg's "Basmati & Wild Rice" blend. Heat a cooking oil, such as the one pictured on this page, to medium heat in a frying pan. Add diced tofu, tempeh <u>or</u> seitan to the pan and while stirring occasionally, fry until golden brown. Once browned, add a little water and then add either shoyu sauce or Bragg's Aminos—about three to six teaspoons, depending on your taste. Simmer for a minute or two. Add beans (any variety) and grated ginger and simmer for two or three minutes. Stir in cut veggies of your choice and prepared grains, stirring frequently. Add Mexican Seasoning or cumin, and add additional shoyu or Bragg's aminos, to taste. Don't overcook the veggies. Scoop onto a plate and add flax oil and Gomasio to taste. Serve with the salad. Very delicious.

Salad Preparation
Salads made with just iceberg lettuce, tomatoes, cabbage and carrots is very old-fashioned, bland and barely nutritious. Salads do NOT have to be boring! Since I always seem to be in a hurry, I often make salads from ingredients I don't have to cut, chop or dice. Besides the traditional salad foods you know about, consider these:

Salad Ingredients (organic, of course)
• Sprouted lentils
• Sprouted garbanzo beans
• Sprouted sunflower seeds
• Sprouted wheat berries
• Mixed leaf greens
• Crimson sprouts
• Cashews
• Pumpkin seeds (try the tamari version too)
• Dried cranberries
• Nutritional yeast
• Flax oil
• Annie's Goddess Dressing

Notice that none of the above ingredients require chopping or cutting—just "grab and drop" onto your plate! It doesn't get much quicker than that, and yet this is a very tasty and nutritious salad. During hot summer months, sometimes I'll make a large salad, and add stir fried tofu, tempeh or seitan. Very nutritious and way better tasting than conventional salads!

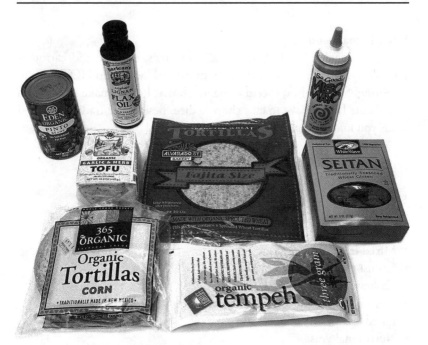

Burritos

Overview
Making the burrito is very similar to making the stir fry. The primary differences are: 1) instead of grains you're using either a flour or corn tortilla, and 2) instead of a salad, you're adding the "alive" food directly to the burrito. Both Mexican Seasoning & cumin work well.

Burrito Preparation
Follow the "stir fry" directions on the previous page, without adding the grains. The shiitake mushrooms can be stir fried at the same time as the faux meat. Once the mixture is browned, add the ginger and the shoyu sauce or aminos (along with a little water). Add beans and Mexican Seasoning or cumin and bring back to a simmer. Adjust the shoyu/aminos and the spice to taste. Add the veggies last and don't overcook. Heat tortilla in a pan (my girlfriend prefers to fry the tortilla in oil to make it crunchy); remove to plate and add cooked food to tortilla. Add any of the "salad ingredients" from the previous page to the tortilla. Add flax oil and

either Annie's Goddess Dressing, or Miso Mayo (pictured—you will find it in the refrigerator section). This is an amazingly delicious and nutritious meal. Mix it up by changing the faux meat (tofu, tempeh or seitan), beans and veggies, and you'll never get bored with this meal! It's my all-time favorite easy-to-prepare meal. [Note that I didn't include salsa, because I rarely eat salsa; however, there are several tasty salsas that can be found in the refrigerator section of the natural food store.]

Veggie Suggestions (Burrito & Stir Fry)
• Shiitake mushrooms (stir fry with the faux meat)
• Ginger—grated (as mentioned earlier)
• Daikon root (a radish)–grated
• Kale (I remove the "spine")
• Red cabbage
• Carrot—grated
• Avocado (or guacamole)

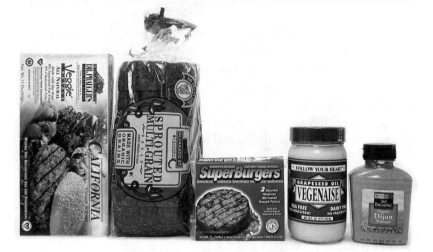

Sandwiches

Overview

A sandwich can be a quick meal to prepare, but by its very nature, it can also be a highly-processed meal—bread, faux meats, dressings, nut butters and jams are all packaged items. Nevertheless, I enjoy eating a sandwich every now and then, and so long as they're consumed in moderation, I think they're fine. The key is to eat all organic so that you maximize nutrition.

Ingredient Options

There are quite a few veggie patty options available at your natural food store. I've tried most of them. Some taste fairly good, though I'm discouraged that so much processing is involved with so many of them. I have found, however, two veggie burgers that I find to be very tasty and minimally processed: Dr. Praegger's veggie burgers (freezer section) and Turtle Island's Super Burgers (refrigerator section). The grapeseed oil Vegenaise by Follow Your Heart is the best mayonnaise substitute I have found. Hummus (not pictured) is an excellent addition to any veggie burger or faux meat sandwich. Although I enjoy Alvarado Street Bakery's bread—which is nationally distributed (freezer or refrigerator)—check to see if there is a local organic bread maker in your area (in your natural food store's bread sec-

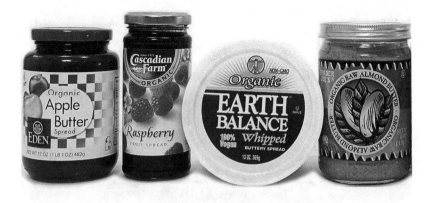

tion); you may be delightfully surprised with the quality. Try raw organic almond butter instead of peanut butter. Eden's apple butter is made without added sugar, which makes it ideal for children. And, of course, notice that virtually every product on this page is made with organic ingredients; try to use only products made with organic ingredients when making sandwiches because there is so little "alive" food in sandwiches.

Sandwich Ingredients Not Pictured
- Avocado
- Tomato
- Sprouts (crimson)
- Faux meats
- Sprouted lentils (delicious on veggie burgers)
- Leaf lettuce

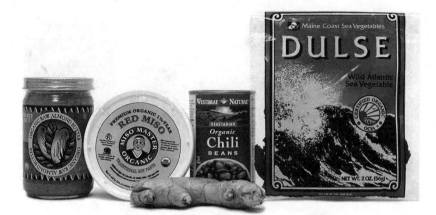

Larry's Morning Miso Soup

The Morning Miso Soup is a very delicious breakfast that I have found to be nourishing, hearty and grounding. This soup is very good for helping people overcome sugar addiction because salt (in the miso paste) is energetically the opposite of sugar. The almond butter adds just enough sweetness to make it a morning meal. I eat this soup for breakfast on a regular basis, and I greatly enjoy it every single time.

In my opinion, this breakfast is far better for you—and especially for children—than cold cereals (even natural) or pancakes/waffles because those foods are too highly processed and contain too much sugar for the morning (e.g. they're too yin/expanding). The other meal I suggest for breakfast is a stir fry—probably with potatoes instead of grains. Both the miso soup and the stir fry are very grounding (yang), making either an ideal breakfast. [See my discussion on yin/yang energy in Chapter 5 for an explanation of how yin and yang foods affect consciousness.]

I had my miso soup served as a breakfast option to film crews in Hollywood, and it was such a hit that every day crew members were asking me for the recipe! Even my finicky nephews like it. So, try the soup and give some to your children. I think you'll find it as delightful as my friends and I do.

The Secret

The secret to this recipe is the almond butter and ginger. You'll always get excellent flavor when you use the ginger/almond butter/miso paste combination. Rotate different veggies and beans in each preparation for variety. If you feel really industrious, cook up some butternut squash, puree it, and add it to the soup (this is *really* delicious!). Enjoy!

Morning Miso Soup Recipe
Makes two bowls of soup.

3 cups water
1/8 cup diced burdock root (very grounding)
1 heaping tablespoon of grated ginger
1/3 cup chopped broccoli
1/4 cup chili beans
1/2 cup chopped kale (high in "B" vitamins)
2 heaping tablespoons of almond butter
1/8 cup grated daikon root (a radish)
1 heaping tablespoon dulse seaweed
2 heaping tablespoons of Miso Master "red" or "barley" miso paste
1 tablespoon flax seed oil

Bring the three cups of water to a boil. Add grated ginger, burdock root and chili beans; bring back to a boil and boil 2 minutes. Turn heat down to medium and add the almond butter. Stir until dissolved, but don't let the water boil over (turn heat lower if you need to). Add kale, broccoli and daikon root. Let cook for about 1 minute, but don't overcook the veggies. Add the seaweed and stir briefly. Turn off burner. Add the miso paste last (and to taste). Miso can easily burn, so don't boil the soup once the miso has been added. Stir the soup until the miso paste is completely dissolved. [Note: Miso Master's "red" miso dissolves faster than the "barley" miso.] Taste the soup. If it is too salty, add water. If it doesn't have enough flavor, add more miso paste (and stir until dissolved). Pour soup into bowls and then add flax oil. Serve with organic toast, if desired. This is my favorite meal of the day.

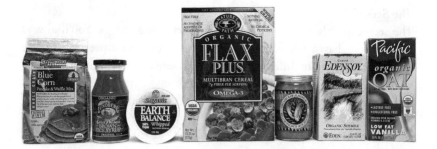

Evening Snack

Overview

As I mentioned on the last page, I believe that cold cereal and pancakes are not suitable for breakfast, primarily because these foods are highly processed and too sweet. Cold cereals and pancakes are a yin food—which means that the energy is expanding—which is better suited to evening than morning. In the morning we want a yang food (contracting, grounding energy), and that means eating cooked foods such as miso soup (as per my recipe) or a breakfast burrito (stir fry some potatoes and follow the burrito recipe). [See my discussion on yin/yang balance in Chapter 5 for more information on the energetics of food.]

As an evening snack, or even a late meal (when you are ready to relax), cold cereal or pancakes can be a delicious, quick and somewhat nutritious meal. I say "somewhat" because typically virtually the entire meal is processed and presented in various packages (cereal, soy milk, pancake mix, buttery spread, etc.), and I'm sure you know by now how much I value eating "alive" food. Nevertheless, I believe it's okay to eat this type of food on occasion, and when you do, again, use products which use only organic ingredients to ensure maximum nutrition. When you eat the products I recommend on this page, you'll find a most delicious blend of flavors suitable to the evening time.

Meal Variations

• Stir almond butter into the cereal and soy milk.
• Try oat milk, and the many other varieties available.
• Try fresh apple juice instead of soy milk.
• Add fresh grated ginger to the pancake batter.
• Add berries to the pancake batter.
• Use Earth Balance buttery spread instead of margarine or butter.
• Instead of using conventionally concocted syrup, try real maple syrup or brown rice syrup—both taste better and are better for you.
• Add berries to your cold cereal.
• Use a nut butter as a pancake topping.
• Buy and eat only 100% organic products of this type, even if other products are labeled "natural."

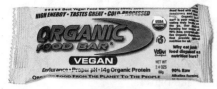 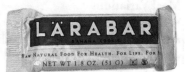

Energy Bars

I work as a location sound mixer on a variety of TV related video productions in Hollywood, California. Quite often we won't get a meal break for five, six or sometimes even eight hours. Thus, I can get pretty hungry and require a boost of energy to keep going for such extended periods of time. I've tried a lot of "energy bars," and by far my two favorites are the "Larabar" and the "Organic Food Bar." Both are made of only whole foods (no highly refined ingredients, such as soy powder), and both are processed at low temperatures, thereby preserving the enzymes. They're both delicious, filling and nutritious. I'm sure you'll find that they meet your expectations.

Resources
Web Sites & Bibliography

I hope that this book has given you the overview you need to confidently begin living a more natural lifestyle. I've tried to touch on most, though not all, topics surrounding the ideals of natural living. As this book is a "beginner's guide," I hope you will further your education as you move forward with this lifestyle. I like to think that the resources I choose are of the highest caliber and integrity, and therefore I feel at ease recommending the following Web sites, and any of the books I have drawn from to write this book.

Organic Consumers Association
www.organicconsumers.org
The *Organic Consumers Association* is an excellent resource for learning more about pesticides/herbicides, irradiation, genetically modified food, mad cow disease and a host of other topics related to food safety.

The Campaign to Label GMO Food
www.thecampaign.org
Upset that you've been lied to in mainstream media about the safety of your food? Then do something about it: help Craig Winters and team pass a law that requires manufacturers of GMO food to label it as such.

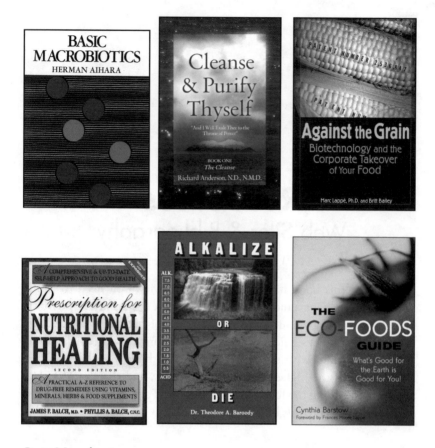

Basic Macrobiotics
    Aihara, Herman (Japan Publications, Inc. 1991)
Cleanse & Purify Thyself
    Anderson, Richard (Anderson, 1994)
Against the Grain
    Bailey, Britt and Lappe, Marc (The Tides Center / CETOS 1998)
Prescription for Nutritional Healing
    Balch, James and Phyllis (Avery Publishing Group 1997)
Alkalize or Die
    Baroody, Theodore (Holographic Health Press 1991)
The Eco-Foods Guide
    Barstow, Cynthia (New Society Publishers 2002)

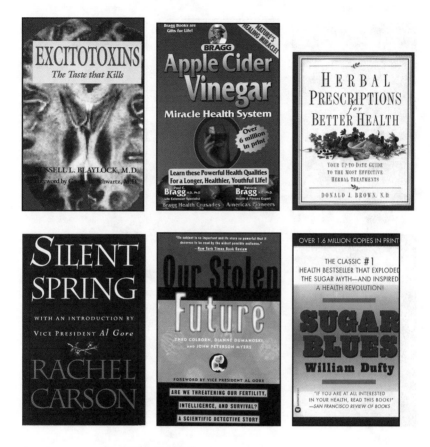

Excitotoxins—The Taste that Kills
    Blaylock, Russell (Health Press 1997)
Apple Cider Vinegar, Miracle Health System
    Bragg, Patricia and Paul (Health Science)
Herbal Prescriptions for Better Health
    Brown, Donald (Prima Publishing 1996)
Silent Spring
    Carson, Rachel (Houghton Mifflin Company 1994)
Our Stolen Future
    Colborn, Theo & Dumanoski, Dianne & Myers, John (PLUME 1997)
Sugar Blues
    Dufty, William (Warner Books 1975)

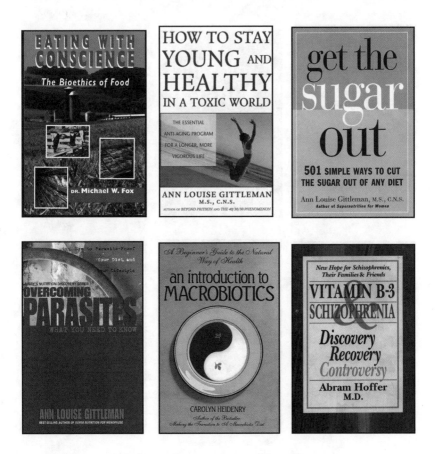

Eating With Conscience
    Fox, Michael (NewSage Press 1997)
How to Stay Young and Healthy in a Toxic World
    Gittleman, Ann Louise (Keats Publishing 1999)
Get the Sugar Out
    Gittleman, Ann Louise (Three Rivers Press 1996)
Overcoming Parasites
    Gittleman, Ann Louise (Avery Publishing Group 1999)
An Introduction to Macrobiotics
    Heidenry, Carolyn (Avery Publishing Group 1992)
Vitamin B-3 & Schizophrenia
    Hoffer, Abram (Quary Press, Inc. 1998)

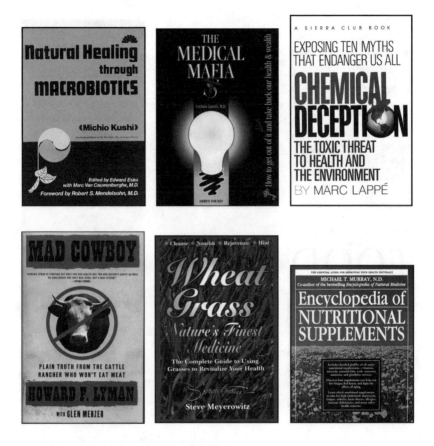

Natural Healing through Macrobiotics
    Kushi, Michio (Japan Publications, Inc. 1978)
The Medical Mafia
    Lanctot, Guylaine (Here's the Key, Inc. 1995)
Chemical Deception
    Lappe, Marc (Sierra Club Books 1991)
Mad Cowboy
    Lyman, Howard (Touchstone 1998)
Wheat Grass – Nature's Finest Medicine
    Meyerowitz, Steve (Sproutman Publications 1999)
Encyclopedia of Nutritional Supplements
    Murray, Michael (Prima Publishing 1996)

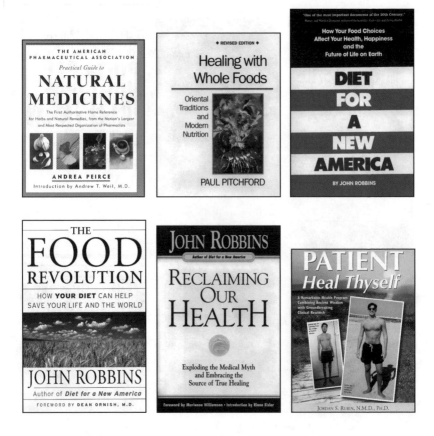

Practical Guide to Natural Medicines
    Peirce, Andrea (The Stonesong Press, Inc. 1999)
Healing with Whole Foods
    Pitchford, Paul (North Atlantic Books 1993)
Diet for a New America
    Robbins, John (Stillpoint Publishing 1987)
The Food Revolution
    Robbins, John (Conari Press 2001)
Reclaiming Our Health
    Robbins, John (HJ Krammer, Inc. 1996)
Patient Heal Thyself
    Rubin, Jordan (Freedom Press 2004)

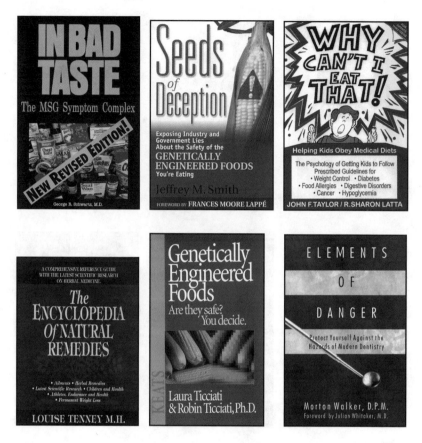

In Bad Taste
    Schwartz, George (Health Press 1999)
Seeds of Deception
    Smith, Jeffrey (YES! Books, 2003)
Why Can't I Eat That!
    Taylor, John F. and Latta, Sharon R. (ADD-Plus 1996)
The Encyclopedia of Natural Remedies
    Tebbey, Louise (Woodland Publishing, Inc. 1995)
Genetically Engineered Foods
    Ticciati, Laura and Robin (Keats Publishing, Inc. 1998)
Elements of Danger
    Walker, Morton (Hamptom Roads Publishing Company, Inc. 2000)

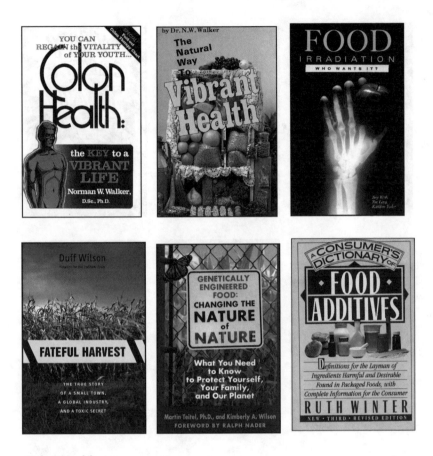

Colon Health
    Walker, Norman (O'Sullivan Woodside & Company 1979)
The Natural Way to Vibrant Health
    Walker, Norman (Norwalk Press 1972)
Food Irradiation
    Webb, Tony/ Lang, Tim/ Tucker, Kathleen (Thorsons Publishers, Inc. 1987)
Fateful Harvest
    Wilson, Duff (HarperCollins 2001)
Genetically Engineered Food: Changing the Nature of Nature
    Wilson, Kimberly (Park Street Press 1999)
A Consumer's Dictionary of Food Additives
    Winter, Ruth (Crown Publishers, Inc. 1989)

Notes

Chapter 1
[1] A study conducted in 1995 by the N.R.D.C. found that 18,500 of the nation's water systems violated safe drinking water laws, affecting some 45 million Americans.
[2] *Organic Style*; September, 2004, p. 112.
[3] *Healing with Whole Foods*, Paul Pitchford, p. 83.
[4] Ibid., p. 87, annotation 9.
[5] *How To Stay Young and Healthy in a Toxic World*, Ann Louise Gittleman, p. 125.
[6] *Prescription for Nutritional Healing*, Second Edition; James F. and Phyllis A. Balch, p. 31.
[7] Fluoride Action Network, www.fluoridealert.org/dental-fluorosis.htm
[8] Fluoride Action Network, www.fluoridealert.org/f-teeth.htm
[9] Fluoride Action Network, www.fluoridealert.org/fluoride-facts.htm
[10] Personal interview with Dr. Gerard F. Judd, Ph.D., chemist, 9/20/02, see http://goodteeth.tripod.com/judd.htm for more information.
[11] Report by GDT Corporation presented October 20, 1998 in Vancouver, Canada to International Ozone Association Pan American Group; study of Sublette, Illinois Hydrozon water treatment system, p. 11.
[12] Available through GAIAM (www.gaiam.com) 877-9896321.
[13] *How To Stay Young and Healthy in a Toxic World*, Ann Louise Gittleman, p. 134.
[14] Custom Pure can also be reached at 206-363-0039 or 1514 NE 179th Street Seattle, WA 98155.
[15] Living Waters is a joint project of the Pacific Rivers Council, American Wildlands and the Yellowstone to Yukon Conservation Initiative (www.pacrivers.org) Phone 541-345-0119.

Chapter 2
Pesticides and Herbicides
[1] Pesticide Watch, http://www.pesticidewatch.org/Html/PestProblem/PestProblem.htm.
[2] Lecture in Washington State on Bainbridge Island, 1998, Howard Lyman, former rancher/farmer, and author of *Mad Cowboy*. Mr. Lyman used to use synthetic pesticides on his farm/ranch and discovered later how poisonous they were, how the worms vanished from his soil and how the soil died. He devotes

his time to exposing this information to the public as well as other health concerns that pertain to diet.

[3] Environmental Toxins and Reproductive Health, http://womenshealth.about.com/health/womenshealth/library/weekly/aa061599.htm?iam=ma.

[4] Environmental Working Group, http://foodnews.org/questions.html#TOXIC (expired link).

[5] Chemical fertilizers have also been found to contain toxic chemicals and poisonous heavy metals such as lead, arsenic and other industrial waste by-products. This is because many synthetic chemical manufacturers have been buying toxic industrial waste from various companies to use in their fertilizers. *This waste usually requires a permit for disposal because of its toxicity to the environment.* This was first brought to the attention of the people in Seattle in 1997 when newspaper columnist Duff Wilson broke the story "Fear in the fields: How hazardous wastes become fertilizer," which ran in the *Seattle Times* on Thursday, July 3, 1997. The story led to investigations and proposed changes in state law. Later, some laws went into effect allowing the practice to continue, provided the toxic chemicals were listed on the Internet so anyone could review them. Mr. Wilson won a literary award for his story. He later wrote a book on the subject: *Fateful Harvest.*

[6] *Eating With Conscience, The Bioethics of Food*, Dr. Michael W. Fox, p. 60.

[7] *Against the Grain – Biotechnology and the Corporate Takeover of Your Food*, Marc Lappe, Ph.D. and Britt Bailey, p. 102; and *Agrow: World Crop Protection News*, 12/13/96.

[8] DDT has been found in virtually every living animal on this planet, from East to West and from North to South. It takes dozens or hundreds of years to break down. It has been linked with human cancer and the death of wildlife.

[9] *Silent Spring*, Rachel Carson, p. 227.

[10] Animal products accumulate these toxins in their fat, and so the accumulated amounts are passed on to those who eat meat.

[11] *Diet For A New America*, John Robbins, p. 321.

[12] Neurotoxicity: Adverse effects on the structure or function of the central and/or peripheral nervous system caused by exposure to a toxic chemical. Symptoms of neurotoxicity include muscle weakness, loss of sensation and motor control, tremors, cognitive alterations and autonomic nervous system dysfunction. http://www.trufax.org/general/chemical.html.

[13] Environmental Working Group. This group does an excellent job of citing their sources of information, often from government agencies.

[14] *Chemical Deception: The Toxic Threat to Health and the Environment*, Marc Lappe, pp. 86-87.

[15] *Eating With Conscience, The Bioethics of Food*, Dr. Michael W. Fox, p. 61;

Washington Post, June 28th, 1993.

[16] *Diet For A New America*, John Robbins, pp. 318.

[17] Ibid., pp. 308-349.

[18] World Wildlife Fund.

[19] Medical doctors, university scholars, environmentalists, etc.

[20] Endocrine Toxicity: Any adverse structural and/or functional changes to the endocrine system (the system that controls hormones in the body) which may result from exposure to chemicals. Endocrine toxicity can harm human and animal reproduction and development. http://www.trufax.org/general/chemical.html.

[21] http://www.pmac.net/erice.htm.

[22] Think about this concept for a moment—wearing rubber gloves because of the pesticides. Does this food sound safe to you?!

[23] Indian Express Newspapers (Bombay) Ltd., http://www.indian-express.com/ie/daily/19971219/35250023.html.

[24] Pest Management at the Crossroads, Benbrook, Consumers Union 1996; "Cancer among farmers: A review," Scand J. Work Environ Health 1985; Our Stolen Future, Theo Colburn.

[25] *Chemical Deception: The Toxic Threat to Health and The Environment*, Marc Lappe, p. 41.

[26] However, there are links to many other chemicals as well. And of course, pesticides and herbicide exposure are not the only causes of disease.

[27] "The Great Boycott," http://home.earthlink.net/~alto/boycott.html (expired link).

[28] Entire paragraph from "Pesticide Watch," http://www.pesticidewatch.org/Html/PestProblem/MythSafety.htm.

Genetically Modified Organisms

[1] *Genetically Engineered Foods – Are They Safe? You Decide*, Laura and Robin Ticciati, p. xi.

[2] *Genetically Engineered Food: Changing the Nature of Nature*, Martin Teitel, Ph.D. and Kimberly A. Wilson, p.17.

[3] Ibid.

[4] Ibid., p.52.

[5] *New Scientist*, 1999.

Irradiation

[1] Virginia Polytechnic Institute, www.ext.vt.edu/pubs/foods/458-300/458-300.html.

[2] Food Irradiation Alert! "An Inside Report on Food Safety and the Food In-

dustry," Aug./Sept. 2001 Vol. 2, No. 4' found at: www.citizen.org/cmep/food-safety/food_irrad/.

[3] Environment News Service and BioDemocracy and Organic Consumers Association, www.purefood.org/irrad/radiodurans.cfm.

[4] Public Citizen, Critical Mass Energy & Environment Program, www.citizen.org.

[5] Ibid.

[6] S.G. Srikantia, B.Sc., B.B.S., D.Sc., Professor of Food and Nutrition, University of Mysore, India; Donald, Louria, Ph.D., Chairman, Department of Preventative Medicine and Community Health, University of Medicine & Dentistry, New Jersey; George Tritsch, Ph.D., Cancer Research Scientist, Rosewell Park Memorial Institute, New York State Department of Health; and Richard Piccioni, Ph.D., Senior Staff Scientist, Accord Research and Educational Associates, New York, NY; http://ccnr.org/food_irradiation.html.

[7] Ibid.

[8] Ibid.

[9] Ibid.

[10] Ibid.

Food Additives

[1] The food-additive industry has been trying to get this law repealed for quite some time now.

[2] Ibid.

[3] The natural foods industry, which typically uses no synthetic chemicals, can often find ways of increasing shelf life through natural means. Nevertheless, shelf life among natural foods is usually less than for mainstream foods. This is one reason why the food costs more. However, paying more for food is better than paying to find a cure for a disease that could have been prevented.

[4] The life force, in the simplest terms, makes a plant grow. Even after a plant has been harvested, its life force will remain—for awhile. This is why it's always a good idea to eat food that's as fresh as possible. It's also why you might have heard about people eating sprouted foods—they're seeking out the energy that the food contains.

[5] *The Goldbecks' Guide to Good Food*, Nikki & David Goldbeck, p. 18.

[6] *The Bread & Circus Whole Food Bible*, Christopher S. Kilham, p. 4.

[7] UBIC: Consultants In Industrial Strategy & Marketing For The Food & Chemical Industries.

[8] *Why Your Child Is Hyperactive*, Ben F. Feingold, (New York: Random House, 1996).

[9] S.J. Schoenthaler, W.E. Doraz, J.A. Wakefield, "The Impact of a Low Food

Additive and Sucrose Diet on Academic Performance in 803 New York City Public Schools," *Int J Biosocial Res.*, 1986, 8(2); pp. 185–195. Quoted by the Feingold Association of the United States.

Aspartame

[1] *The Psycho-Social, Chemical, Biological and Electromagnetic Manipulation of Human Consciousness*, Val Valerian, Leading Edge Research Group, p. 138.

[2] Excitotoxin: a substance added to foods and beverages that literally stimulates neurons to death, causing brain damage of varying degrees.

[3] Aspartame Kills Web site, www.aspartame.com/blalockpilot.htm.

[4] Ralph G. Walton, M.D., Chairman, The Center for Behavioral Medicine, Professor and Chairman, Department of Psychiatry, Northeastern Ohio Universities College of Medicine; DORway, www.dorway.com/peerrev.html.

[5] Information for last three paragraphs: "Could There Be Evils Lurking In Aspartame Consumption?", Christine Lydon, MD, *OXYGEN MAGAZINE*, October issue; reprinted at Aspartame Kills, www.aspartamekills.com/lydon.htm.

[6] Aspartame Consumer Safety Network.

[7] Dr. Marvin Legator, Director of Environmental Toxicology at the University of Texas, who helped pioneer the mutagecity testing at the FDA, is quoted as saying, "All of Searle tests are scientifically irresponsible and disgraceful," and on April 8th, 1976, Senator Edward Kennedy, a member of the Senate Subcommittee that oversaw an investigation into aspartame and other drugs of Searle, stated, "The extensive nature of the almost unbelievable ranges of abuses discovered by the FDA on several major Searle products is profoundly disturbing." *The Psycho-Social, Chemical, Biological and Electromagnetic Manipulation of Human Consciousness,* Val Valerian, Leading Edge Research Group, pp. 152-153.

[8] *The Psycho-Social, Chemical, Biological and Electromagnetic Manipulation of Human Consciousness,* Val Valerian, Leading Edge Research Group, p. 138.

[9] "Aspartame, The Condoned Lethal Sweetener," by Phil Macdonald, *The Latest Magazine,* reprinted at DORway: www.dorway.com/lethal.html.

[10] *The Psycho-Social, Chemical, Biological and Electromagnetic Manipulation of Human Consciousness,* Val Valerian, Leading Edge Research Group, p. 155.

[11] Pages S5507 through S5511 of the Congressional Record dated May 7, l985; DORway, www.dorway.com/nsda.html.

Sugar

[1] *The Psycho-Social, Chemical, Biological and Electromagnetic Manipulation of Human Consciousness*, Val Valerian, p. 127 (www.trufax.org).

[2] *Get the Sugar Out*, Ann Louise Gittleman, page xxvii.

[3] www.princeton.edu/pr/news/02/q2/0620-hoebel.htm.

[4] *Michigan Organic News*, William Code Martin, March 1957.
[5] www.monsanto.com/monsanto/layout/media/00/03-27-00.asp.

Refined Oils and Salt
[1] *Health Food Labels May Deceive*, Dr. Dane Roubos, B.Sc., D.C., www.whale.
to/a/roubos.html
[2] *The Healing Miracles of Coconut Oil*, Bruce Fife, N.D., www.thepowermall.
com/thecenterforhealth/bio/fife.htm
[3] *Healing With Whole Foods*, Paul Pitchford, p. 141.
[4] *Basic Macrobiotics*, Herman Aihara, p. 59.
[5] *Healing With Whole Foods*, Paul Pitchford, pp. 156-162.

Monosodium Glutamate (MSG)
[1] *In Bad Taste–The MSG Symptom Complex*, George R. Schwartz, M.D., p. 2.
[2] Ibid., p. 61
[3] *The Feel Good Handbook*, Annie Costa, The Lighthouse Press, http://thelight-housepress.com.
[4] Experimental studies show that glutamate acts as a trigger that opens the sodium channel on the cell membrane and allows calcium to enter the neuron, triggering an enzyme called phospholipase C within the cell, which then triggers the release of arachidonic acid, damaging the cell's interior. The arachidonic acid is attacked by two enzymes called lipoygenase and cyclo-oxygenase, further triggering an explosive release of free radicals (superoxide and hydroxyl radicals) which brings on cell death. The normal concentration of antioxidants in the brain is not enough to handle the excess free radicals produced in this way. The Leading Edge Research Group, www.trufax.org.
[5] www.nomsg.com - Hidden Sources.
[6] *In Bad Taste – The MSG Symptom Complex*, George R. Schwartz, M.D., p. 9.
[7] *In Bad Taste – The MSG Symptom Complex*, George R. Schwartz, M.D., p. 13; Federation Proceedings, April 1977.
[8] *The Feel Good Handbook*, Annie Costa, The Lighthouse Press, http://thelight-housepress.com.
[9] Society for Neuroscience 19th Annual Meeting, Phoenix, Arizona, October, 1989; *The Psycho-Social, Chemical, Biological and Electromagnetic Manipulation of Human Consciousness*, Val Valerian, Leading Edge Research Group, p. 175.
[10] Science Service Report 1993, studies by James Golomb of New York University.
[11] "Excitotoxin Food Additives: Functional Teratological Aspects," Dr. John Onley, *Progressive Brain Research, Vol. 18*, 1988, p. 283.

Chapter 6

[1] *Healing With Whole Foods*, Paul Pitchford, pp. 188-189.
[2] *Wheat Grass—Nature's Finest Medicine*, Steve Meyerowitz, p. 23.
[3] *Healing With Whole Foods*, Paul Pitchford, page 529.
[4] Ibid., p. 191.
[5] *Encyclopedia of Nutritional Supplements*, Michael T. Murray, N.D., pp. 359-364; *The Encyclopedia of Natural Remedies*, Louise Tenney, M.H., pp. 176-177; "Probiotics Balance Digestion & Improve Overall Health," Anthony Cichoke, D.C. (reprint), *Nutrition Science News*, August 1997, pp. 380-382.
[6] *Encyclopedia of Nutritional Supplements*, Michael T. Murray, N.D., pp. 249-268.
[7] *Prescription for Nutritional Healing*, by James Balch and Phyllis Balch, p. 51.
[8] *Fresh Vegetable and Fruit Juices—What's Missing in Your Body?*, N.W. Walker, p. 65.
[9] *Apple Cider Vinegar – Miracle Health System*, Paul C. and Patricia Bragg, N.D., Ph.D. See www.bragg.com.

Chapter 7

[1] *Cleanse & Purify Thyself*, Dr. Richard Anderson, N.D., N.M.D., p. 10.

Chapter 8

[1] Dennis Hughes Interviews Jack LaLanne 2001, The Share Guide, *The Holistic Health Magazine*.

Chapter 9

[1] From *The Way of* chigong, *the Art and Science of Chinese Energy Healing*, Kenneth S. Cohen.

Chapter 10

[1] *The Medical Mafia*, Guylaine Lanctot, M.D., p. 35.
[2] Ibid., p. 33.
[3] Ibid.; Additional information on Flexner can be found here: www.unmc.edu/Community/ruralmeded/flexner.htm.
[4] *The Medical Mafia*, Guylaine Lanctot, M.D., p. 37.
[5] *Reclaiming Our Health*, John Robbins, p. 188.
[6] Ibid., p. 193.
[7] Ibid. pages 273-278
[8] William Morrow and Co., Inc. 1995

Chapter 11

[1] In the September 1997 *Journal of British Medicine*, research showed that there can be a causal relationship between periodontal disease and an increase in heart problems. In some of the populations studied, the likelihood of getting heart disease doubled when periodontal problems are present.

[2] German doctors Voll, Kramer, Adler, Gleditch, Rau and others found that relationships and body maps exist in the mouth; these researchers developed charts to help practitioners relate dental disease to distant sites in the body.

[3] www.altcorp.com/AffinityLaboratory/toxicvsinfected.htm.

[4] Endocal© is available to dentists through Biodent in Montreal.

[5] Calcium hydroxide is ultimately converted to calcium carbonate, creating a wall of calcification at vital tissue, sealing root apices and vital dentin tubules. Calcium hydroxide is also more effective than paramonochlorophenol (PMCP), a commonly used root canal medication, in killing anaerobic bacteria associated with infected root canals.

[6] The American Dental Association estimates that 75% of those over twenty have some form of periodontal disease.

[7] See *Elements of Danger*, Morton Walker, DPM, pps. 299-301 for a comprehensive list of specific supplements suggested for healing periodontal disease.

[8] Prickly ash bark has been studied in medical/dental research and has been shown to possess antiseptic, disinfectant and deodorant properties, according to Robert Arthur, DDS, of Santa Barbara, CA.

[9] You can get MistORAL from Brower Enterprises, Inc. (800-373-6076) or brower.ent@dtg.net.com . To obtain the NDHM&GT product, call Woodstock Natural Products ("The Natural Dentist" at 8000-615-6895) or natdent@worldnet.att.net.

Conclusion

[1] Except for occasional salmon in the last two years.

About The Author

Author and publisher Larry Cook became a passionate advocate for natural living after reading John Robbins' revolutionary book *Diet for a New America*. The book changed his life – he became a vegetarian, lost 40 pounds and had more energy than ever before. Larry's success with this lifestyle and subsequent years of research inspired him to publish two magazines devoted to natural living. He hired writers to create custom articles on a wide variety of topics he was passionate about, including the manipulation of our food supply, natural medicine, holistic dentistry and environmental toxins, to name a few.

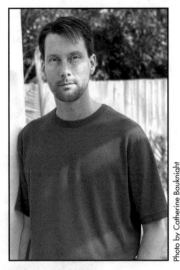

Photo by Catherine Bauknight

The *Natural Life News & Directory*, launched in 2000, now boasts a circulation of 12,000 in Bozeman, Montana, and *The EcoVision Journal* – launched in 2001 – enjoyed a wide, loyal readership in Seattle, Washington until it was sold in 2002. In both cities the magazines became a trusted authority on health, environmental and other natural lifestyle issues.

Larry co-wrote, with Deborah Merlin, **Victory Over ADHD**: *How a mother's journey to natural medicine reversed her children's severe emotional, mental and behavioral problems*. The book shares Deborah's heart wrenching story of her dysfunctional twins and how she ultimately turned to natural medicine to do what conventional medicine couldn't, and Larry shares insights backed by research as to the multiple causes and cures for ADD/ADHD. It's available from www.VictoryOverADHD.com, www. Amazon.com and your local health food store or bookstore.

Larry studied video/film production and photography at Clover Park Vocational-Technical Institute in Tacoma, Washington, and received his bachelor's degree from The Evergreen State College in Olympia, Washington. In addition to serving as a tireless advocate for natural living, Larry is a photographer and works in video/film production in Los Angeles.

Order Information

To order additional copies of this book please go to:

www.TheNaturalGuide.com or **www.Amazon.com**

Also by Larry Cook

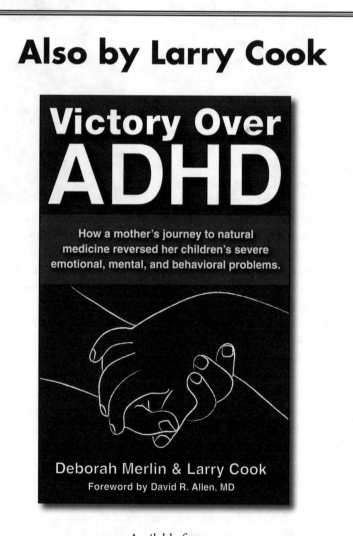

Available from:

www.VictoryOverADHD.com or **www.Amazon.com**